101

WAYS TO BURN FAT

ON THE BALL

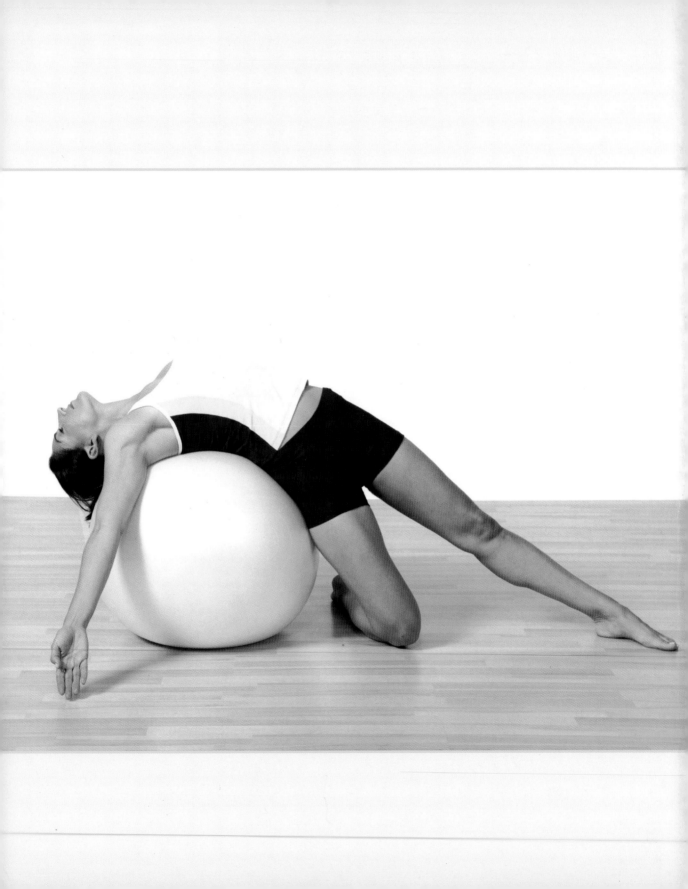

101
WAYS TO BURN FAT
ON THE BALL

Lose Weight with Fun Cardio and Body-Sculpting Moves!

LIZBETH GARCIA

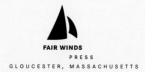

FAIR WINDS
PRESS
GLOUCESTER, MASSACHUSETTS

Text © 2006 by Lizbeth Garcia

First published in the USA in 2006 by
Fair Winds Press, a member of
Quayside Publishing Group
33 Commercial Street
Gloucester, MA 01930

10 09 08 07 06   2 3 4 5

ISBN - 13: 978-1-59233-207-6
ISBN - 10: 1-59233-207-2

Library of Congress Cataloging-in-Publication Data

Garcia, Lizbeth.

  101 ways to burn fat on the ball: lose weight with fun cardio and body-
sculpting moves! / Lizabeth Garcia.

     p. cm.

  ISBN 1-59233-207-2

  1. Medicine balls. 2. Exercise. I. Title: One hundred one ways to burn fat
on the ball. II. Title: One hundred and one ways to burn fat on the ball. III.
Title.

  GV496.G55 2006

  613.7'1--dc22

Cover and book design by *Laura H. Couallier, Laura Herrmann Design*
Photography by *Allan Penn*
Hair cut and color by *Lisa Moore at C13 Salon, San Diego*
Manicure and pedicure by *Pamela Couch at Gila Rut Salon, San Diego*

Printed and bound in Singapore

The information in this book is for educational purposes only. It is not
intended to replace the advice of a physician or medical practitioner. Please
see your health care provider before beginning any new health program.

This book is dedicated to my family,
Mirta, Francisco, and Gabriel.

To my husband, Pete Tillack,
and our loving parents Sue and Geoff of Sydney, Australia.

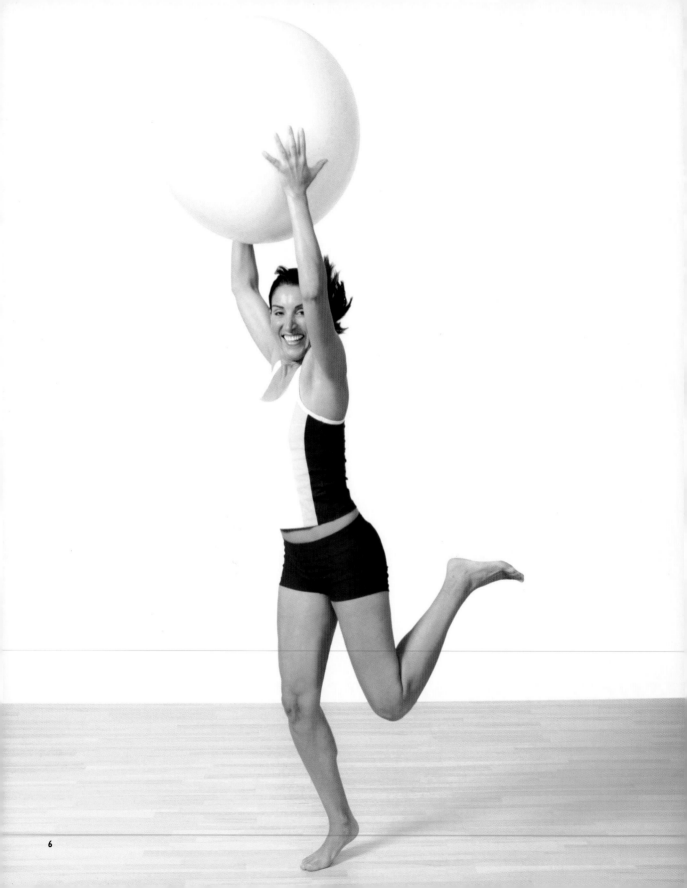

Contents

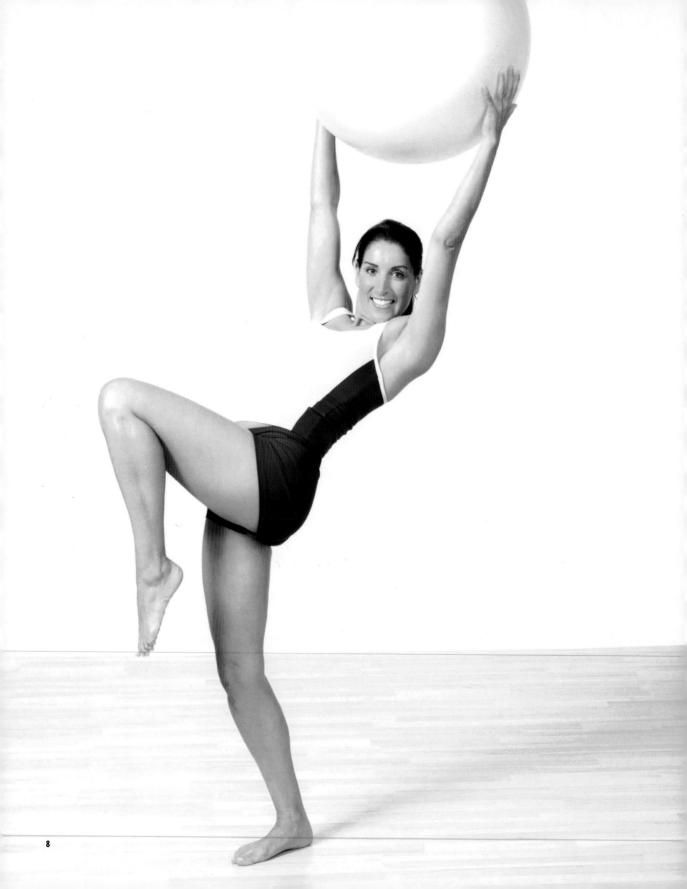

The Ball:
The Best Fitness Tool Around

The treadmill. The Step. The elliptical trainer. Yoga. Pilates. Over the 15 years I've been working out regularly and teaching exercise, only a few things have revolutionized the fitness world. That's because no matter what type of exercise you do, the basic truths and equations of weight loss and health are always the same: Get your heart rate up at least a few times a week for cardiovascular health and to burn any excess calories, do strength training to keep your muscles strong and your body toned, and use some form of mind-body exercise to relax your muscles and stay in touch with your spirit.

The ball hasn't changed those truths—it doesn't magically burn calories or strengthen your muscles without you even trying. Nevertheless, I consider the ball to be nothing short of a miracle because it reinvigorated the same old exercises—including the ones I mentioned above—such as strength training, yoga, and Pilates. The ball is inexpensive and easy to use and yet it can challenge even the most advanced exerciser in a seemingly endless number of ways.

Let me show you what I mean. Let's take, for example, one of the most common—and effective—moves, the squat. Doing a squat is fairly easy, you just have to pretend you're sitting in a chair. Just doing that move strengthens your quadriceps (the front of your thighs), gluteals (your butt), and your hamstrings (the backs of your thighs). It's also beneficial for your abdominals and lower legs, too. And here's another benefit: the squat uses the large muscles of your butt and legs so it also burns a nice number of calories if you do enough of them.

How can the ball make this move even more effective (and fun)? Well, here are just a few ways: If you're a beginning exerciser, you can use the ball as a guide and put it beneath you as you squat. Or, another option is to put the ball against the wall and roll against it as you sink into your squat. And here are two more ideas: hold the ball in front of your chest as you squat to add resistance to the move (which will tone your upper body and burn more calories) or, to make the squat even tougher, hold the ball above your head.

But I forgot one very important squat alternative—you can actually just sit on the ball and bounce if you're really not yet in the kind of shape that allows you to do a real squat. Even sitting and bouncing on the ball tones your muscles because you have to contract muscles to stay on top of a round seat.

So, as you can see, the ball has something to offer everyone. Because of its versatility, it's an especially great tool for someone like me—a personal trainer and group exercise instructor—because it allows me to be creative and have fun when I'm teaching and helping someone get into shape.

Expect the Unexpected

I created this program to keep the body moving, but one of its greatest benefits is spontaneity. Each time I start a class, my students don't really know what to expect. Of course they know we are going to move a lot and we're going to use the ball for every move, whether cardio or resistance, but what they don't know is the order in which we are going to do the steps and moves and which variations of the moves we are going to do.

That's why I decided to put 101 moves in this book. Of course, you won't do 101 moves each time you work out, but once you're familiar with the moves in the thirty-minute and sixty-minute workouts, you'll be able to mix and match some of your favorite moves and routines to create your perfect workouts.

I also created ten short, targeted programs that will benefit you in two ways. First, if you're pressed for time or have a specific body-shaping concern, then you can use these routines to reach your goals. Second, you can use these moves to help create your own thirty-minute or longer workouts.

Changing up your routines not only helps your workout stay fresh and fun, but it also helps make you fit faster. Here's why: your muscles can actually get into a fitness rut, so if you only regularly walk three miles in 45 minutes or if you only lift two-pound dumbbells and do the same eight exercises during every workout, eventually what was once a challenging program will be a boring and easy series of movements for your body. Now, hardcore muscle builders simply increase the amount of weight they use to continue challenging their bodies. The results of that type of training are stronger and bigger muscles, but that's not the goal for most of us. Most of us just want to get fit and stay that way. So, in order to keep challenging our muscles, we can simply surprise them with new exercises and new routines. This way, our muscles will never get used to the program we're doing.

A Workout That "Doesn't Seem Like Work"

The regulars in my class include Danielle Dorman, 37, mother of two seven-year-old twins, who says "exercising on the ball doesn't seem like work. I love the music and the environment and it is a very vigorous workout." Danielle has lost at least ten pounds since taking my "On the Ball Pilates" class. "I have better posture, more core strength, and more awareness of my form and intention when I lift weights or do other forms of exercise," Danielle adds. "And I love how versatile the ball is—I can use it for strength training, stretching, aerobics, and almost anything else."

Let me just tell you a little more about the fitness ball before I tell you how we're going to use it. The ball has been around the exercise world for years, but only recently have personal trainers started to find ways to lift weights and practice yoga and Pilates with it. But as great as strength training and yoga and Pilates are, for many people, exercise is all about burning fat. Of course, you need muscle to burn fat (I'll explain why in a minute) but for many of us, exercise feels best when we're moving and dancing with our whole body.

Why The Ball is Such a Great Tool

When you stand with both feet on the ground you have a few things helping you keep your balance: First, the ground is steady. Second, your feet are designed to hold you upright. When you sit on the ball, however, those two elements are taken away. The ball is an unsteady surface so your body has to keep itself upright by using other muscles to hold its weight. Furthermore, most of us don't use those balancing or "core" muscles enough to keep them strong and functional.

KERI DAVIS, 40, Business Owner, Motivational Speaker
Gila Rut Salon, San Diego, CA

Fourteen years ago, I started my own company. Today, my business is soaring and for the past several years I have presented motivational seminars all over the United States.

In mid-2004, I looked in the mirror and saw the thirty-nine-year-old, 222.5-pound woman I had become. I thought it would be a good time to start working out and get in shape. So, I called one of my sister's friends, Lizbeth Garcia, who I knew was a personal trainer. I asked Lizbeth for help and guidance with a fitness and nutrition plan. She provided me with both. The plan was for me to cut my calories and workout with Lizbeth two to three times a week and on my own an additional three to four times a week.

Fast-forward to five months later—December 2004. I hadn't really stayed on plan. If I am honest (and what's the point in not being honest with myself), my diet hadn't changed much and I was only working out when I met with Lizbeth. I became frustrated and began surrendering to the idea that I was destined to be a women's size 20. Who knew—maybe God made me this size so I wouldn't spend too much money on clothes.

As January 2005 approached, my thoughts turned to my fortieth birthday approaching in February. Around that time, some things began to change! That something were my thoughts and my attitude. After seeing Oprah transition herself in her fiftieth year and watching the television show *The Biggest Loser,* it finally hit me...there is no magic pill... there is no magic solution. If I wanted to be healthy, fit, and feel great, I had to make the decision that I was committed to attaining these things.

A TRANSFORMATION

By January 1, 2005, I had made the decision. I resolved to being committed to my own transformation. I made a conscious decision to change and I committed myself to creating that change. I stopped putting things (imaginary and real) in front of my health and my well-being. Instead, I moved these things to the top of my list—every day, with every decision and every action. The first thing I did was to call Lizbeth and recommit myself to six days a week of workouts with her. I then rearranged my work schedule to accommodate this schedule. Lizbeth designed a program for me that coupled cardio-vascular workouts with circuit training. After I built my strength, we started incorporating Pilates and swimming. (Believe it or not, I sometimes work out twice a day!) The other thing I did was to figure out a healthy, low-fat food plan that worked for me, long term. While that plan has evolved, what remains constant is my knowledge that I must constantly balance between calories in and calories out to lose and maintain my weight.

THE RESULTS

I am thrilled to report that my commit-ment to myself and to change, coupled with hard work and persistence, has lead to real results! Eleven months into my new lifestyle, I am a beautiful forty-year-old, 175-pound, size 12 wearing woman! I have lost a total of 42 inches. And I am still going strong! Lizbeth and I reach new goals every day. Today I ran five miles (yep—all at one time—without stopping)! It was my longest run ever. Who knows, maybe next week it will be six miles or even seven! What I do know is that I am capable of whatever I decide I am capable of—and that change starts with that decision. If I can change, you can too!!!! But recently, I became aware of the fact that I had an underlying belief that my power came from my size (5'9" and 222.5 pounds). I thought that my size made me more effective and that if my weight was gone, I wouldn't be as dynamic and successful. I was wrong! I have learned that my power comes from inside; it comes from the inner confidence of knowing that I can do anything I put my mind to. This awareness and my decision to change the way I thought about myself, and the choices I made around exercise and nutrition, has been the biggest accomplishment of my life. If I can change, you can too!!

So when you sit on the ball your body uses muscles that are often weak and under-utilized. Interestingly, these core muscles not only help us with our overall body strength, they also help us look longer and leaner the stronger they are.

The core muscles consist of muscles arranged in layers that not only stabilize your spine but allow it to move. Your deepest abdominal muscle, the transversus abdominis or transverse, provides a girdle of support for your spine by wrapping low around your waist, just as a seatbelt would.

The multifidus is a long and deep muscle running from the sacrum to the cervical vertebrae. The multifidus' primary duty is to stabilize your spine and assist with extension (arching) and rotation (twisting).

The pelvic floor muscles assist in pelvic and spinal stability. Collectively, your pelvic floors make a sling or hammock of muscles that run in two different directions— from your pubic bone to tailbone and from one butt-bone to the other—to support the weight of your organs. In every exercise, you will strive to engage your deep stabilizing muscle—imagine pulling up through your pelvic floors deep within your center and pulling in your bellybutton.

You can feel your belly pull in when your transverse engages around your waist, but the contraction of the multifidus is more subtle. You can feel the pelvic floors engage by stopping the flow of your urine; it's a lift between your legs similar to Kegel exercises. Ideally, lifting the pit of your abdomen should be a soft action (nothing forced or strained).

Several other important muscles form the multiple layers making up your core. These include your internal oblique and your external oblique muscles. These muscles allow you to twist and bend at the waist. The rectus abdominis is a long, shallow abdominal muscle extending from your pubic bone to your sternum. You can feel it engage as you bend forward at the waist. The back muscles are primarily responsible for the extension of the spine. One of the most well-known is the erector spinae; it runs from the sacrum to the last two thoracic vertebrae, helping to extend your spine.

My students love the ball because without a lot of extra exercising, they gain abdominal strength and improve their back flexibility. The ball helps the back muscles (the erector spinae) get stronger and more flexible, which is important for overall back health. If your back muscles are strong, they won't strain when you lift something heavy. Likewise, if your back muscles are flexible then they won't get pulled when you turn around suddenly or reach up high to get something down from a cabinet.

The ball helps all athletes. It was first used in physiotherapy to help injured people gain strength in their stabilizing muscles, because they are so important for allowing us to stand properly. And while injured men and women have used it for simple exercises, athletes (under the direction of their personal trainers) began to use the ball

○ FRANCES PETERSON, 36, Philanthropist

La Jolla, CA

66 **I** haven't had a regimen of exercises since high school, but I have a good time while working out with Lizbeth. She makes it easy to follow her instructions. It takes a lot of effort but I love the results I see in myself. I have tried Pilates a few times with another instructor at another studio and did not get much out of it.

These days I have increased stamina, better posture, and a thinner waist. I now see abs that I didn't see before! I like how I feel after the classes. I get a great physical workout on the ball. It is fun while toning all my muscle groups. Balancing my body on the ball is difficult but I get better at it with every class."

as a challenge tool—it's much harder to do any move, whether it's a bicep curl or a ball toss, when you are trying to balance on the ball.

I've developed classes for exercisers of all levels and types. I hold "On the Ball Pilates" classes as well "Surfers on the Ball" workshops. Think about it: surfers need their core muscles to pull themselves up onto the most unstable surface there is: water.

But it's not just surfers and dance lovers who enjoy my classes. Sylvia Wechter (seventy years old, volunteer, homemaker, psychotherapist) has been a yoga student for many years and now studies Pilates. She finds the ball to be an "innovative way of awakening my body and stretching muscles. Also, I feel secure in not injuring myself. I've noticed an improvement in my muscle tone and am more aware of using my breath to facilitate the exercises. The ball is fun as well as challenging, and an accessible form of exercise."

My Story

I believe that exercising is a positive choice we make for ourselves. It's our daily dosage of natural medicine that makes us feel better, look better, and live longer. Exercise, to me, is another word for living healthy. Your body's health is your choice: choose to exercise and it will help you gain strength, flexibility, balance, stamina, and maintain the quality of your life as you age.

I'm fortunate because I grew up in a family who exercised regularly. In fact, my father and mother have been exercising ever since I can remember. My dad introduced my brother and me to running laps at the track, racquetball and handball, and weight training. The Garcia family joined the local Jack LaLanne gym when it opened on 3rd Avenue in Chula Vista, California. My dad is now sixty-eight and lives with arthritis, but exercise is part of his daily life. He still strength trains, rides the stationary bike, and enjoys his daily steam followed by a freezing cold shower. He walks into the gym with discomfort and pain and walks out feeling good. Exercise is my father's natural medicine.

My mother is now sixty-one and she has been a bilingual educator for the past twenty-five years. She endorses fitness to her elementary school students. My mother's determination to make sure I was able to attend dance class and rehearsals, making handmade costumes for me, and watching from afar in the audience, always made me feel full of love and proud to be in the spotlight. I was her "star in the moment."

Meanwhile, I took dance classes as a little girl that helped me develop self-confidence, poise, and posture. I continued dancing throughout my teens and in college, and added hi- and low-aerobics, running, swimming, and surfing to my active lifestyle. I spent hours on the beach when I wasn't performing in San Diego's Balboa Park yearly dance performance.

As an adult, I became a personal trainer, group exercise instructor, and fitness model. I worked at Rancho La Puerta spa in Tecate, Mexico, and then starred in Harper's Bazaar magazine video "The Bottom Line." Working at Rancho La Puerta helped me learn how to teach, and help people train their bodies, and change their lives.

I also worked at The Golden Door Spa Resort in Escondido, California, was featured in a "Total Ab Roller" infomercial, "Flatten Your Belly with Pilates" a video for Prevention magazine, "The Quick Fix's Abs Pilates," and recently starred in "Cardio Party Mix" for Crunch Fitness.

To keep my energy up and my body fit, I take short breaks to snack on foods that are quick and easy, such as hard-boiled eggs, yogurt, cottage cheese, raw almonds, celery with peanut butter, and fresh fruit. I also take a break for lunch—a salad with tuna, chicken, or beef. I usually have fruit for dessert. Finally, I drink water, hot and cold green tea, and for a quick boost of energy, I put Emer'gen-C in my water, which also adds vitamins and fizz.

When I'm not teaching classes, I enjoy surfing, running, and weight training. I try to do something outside every day of the week for fun.

JAMES PETERSON, 43, Business Executive
La Jolla, CA

"I used to play tennis on a regular basis years ago. I have taken three yoga classes in the past twenty years. I get an effective and complete body workout while having fun in Lizbeth's class and I also really enjoy her style of teaching. She is extraordinarily patient and that is very important to beginners as I was four months ago. Her instructions are precise and easy to follow.

I have increased self-discipline, improved dexterity, and greater self-esteem. My wife says my posture is so much better than before I started the classes. I now see muscle definition where I did not before. Prior to the classes, my body fat was above 19.5%. Four months later, it is below 17% and I have not even changed my eating habits!

I love the exercises on the ball! While balancing and lifting weights, I have to use more coordination with my mind and body. I have ADD and this is a great way to help me focus and stay on track throughout the day."

"I recommend this class to anyone and everyone!"

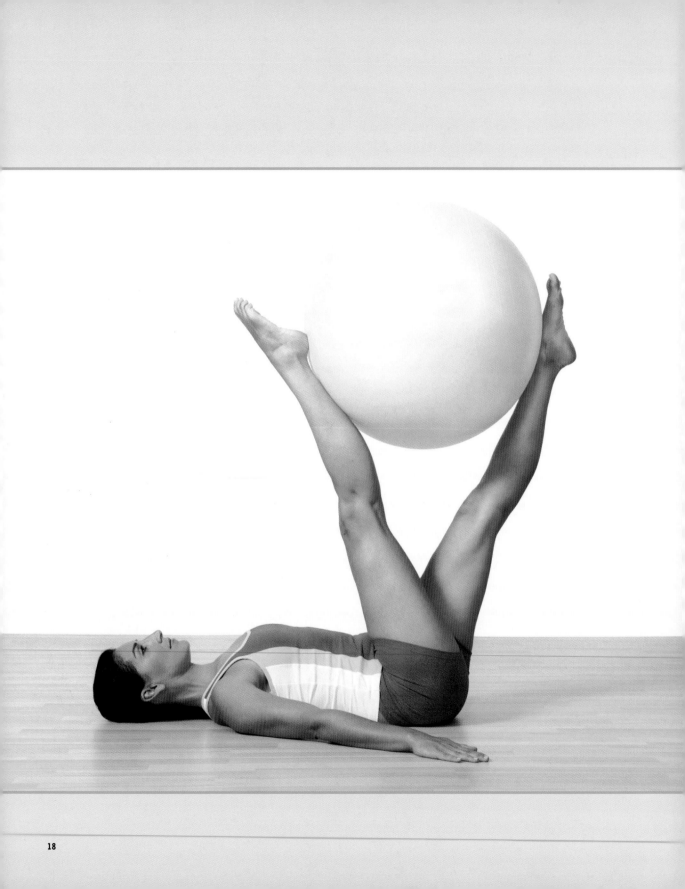

Fat-Burning Secrets

Burning fat is not just a matter of doing more exercise—although that certainly helps. If you're struggling to lose weight, I'm going to explain in great detail exactly what you need to do.

Excess body fat harms the body in a number of ways. First, and most importantly, excess body fat forces the heart to work harder than it is designed to work. The heart muscle works best (i.e., it pumps more easily and forcefully) when someone is the proper weight, because, like an engine, it is of a size relative to the body it lives in. For example, you wouldn't put a Mini Cooper–sized engine in a sixteen-wheel truck and the same is true for a heart.

Overweight people and obese people have a higher incidence of cardiovascular disease than others. The excess weight contributes to high blood pressure (because the heart has to pump harder than it is supposed to in order to move the blood through an over-fat body) and atherosclerosis (fat actually accumulates in the lining of the arterial wall, making the blood vessels thinner and forcing the heart to work even harder than usual to pump blood).

Like the heart, the lungs also have to work overtime in a person who isn't the proper weight. This is why out of shape and over-fat people become winded when they climb stairs or try to take part in athletic activities. Their heart and lungs together cannot manage the excess weight.

Over-fat and overweight people also have a higher incidence of joint problems, because, again, like the heart and lungs, your joints are designed in proportion with the rest of your body; they function best when they only have to carry a proper load.

Systemically, over-fat and overweight people also have a higher incidence of type 2 diabetes, an illness that is often caused by being overweight and over-fat. See the sidebar "Exercise, Diabetes, and Insulin Resistance" for more information.

The real issue though, isn't weight, it is fat. Too much body fat is a health hazard, as much as, if not more than, smoking (the jury is actually still out on which one of these two public health issues causes more deaths each year). And one thing that fights fat is exercise. Exercise—especially resistance exercise—creates muscle, which makes

○ EXERCISE, DIABETES, AND INSULIN RESISTANCE

Over the past few years, diabetes and insulin resistance have become somewhat of an epidemic in the United States and other Western, developed countries. Most researchers and physicians believe that the combination of non-nutritious, high-calorie diets and a lack of physical activities have caused the high incidence of these problems.

Insulin resistance is a silent condition that increases the chances of developing diabetes and heart disease. Learning about insulin resistance is the first step you can take toward making lifestyle changes that will help you prevent diabetes and other health problems. I call it a silent condition because you feel tired and lack energy but you don't know why.

After you eat, the food is broken down into glucose, the simple sugar that is the main source of energy for the body's cells. But your cells cannot use glucose without insulin, a hormone produced by the pancreas. Insulin helps the cells take in glucose and convert it to energy. When the pancreas does not make enough insulin or the body is unable to use the insulin that is present, the cells cannot use glucose. Excess glucose builds up in the bloodstream, setting the stage for diabetes.

Being obese or overweight affects the way insulin works in your body. Extra fat tissue can make your body resistant to the action of insulin, but exercise can help counteract that resistance and help insulin work well.

If you have insulin resistance, your muscle, fat, and liver cells do not use insulin properly. The pancreas tries to keep up with the demand for insulin by producing more. Eventually, the pancreas cannot keep up with the body's need for insulin, and excess glucose builds up in the bloodstream. Many people with insulin resistance have high levels of blood glucose and high levels of insulin circulating in their blood at the same time.

People with blood glucose levels that are higher than normal but not yet in the diabetic range have "pre-diabetes." If you have pre-diabetes, you have a higher risk of developing type 2 diabetes, formerly called adult-onset diabetes or noninsulin-dependent diabetes. Studies have shown that most people with pre-diabetes go on to develop type 2 diabetes within ten years unless they lose 5 to 7 percent of their body weight—which is about ten to fifteen pounds for someone who weighs 200 pounds—by making modest changes in their diet and level of physical activity. People with pre-diabetes also have a higher risk of heart disease.

Type 2 diabetes is sometimes defined as the form of diabetes that develops when the body does not respond properly to insulin, as opposed to type 1 diabetes, in which the pancreas makes no insulin at all. With type 2, the pancreas initially is able to keep up with the added demand by producing more insulin. In time, however, it loses the ability to secrete enough insulin in response to meals.

Because insulin resistance tends to run in families, we know that genes are partly responsible. Excess weight also contributes to insulin resistance because too much fat interferes with muscles' ability to use insulin. Lack of exercise further reduces muscles' ability to use insulin.

One important solution to all of these problems is, of course, exercise. Exercise strengthens the heart (by training it to pump blood effectively) and the lungs (by increasing its capacity), and it builds joint and bone health through impact exercise. Exercise is not the only solution to these problems—you do need to eat well and practice stress management and other healthy habits—but many physicians do consider exercise to be so effective and important that it has been called a "magic bullet"—it is a cure for many illnesses and conditions.

Exercise—which usually means a raised heart rate and muscle movement of a raised intensity (in plain English, this means you're breathing heavy and your muscles are working harder than they do at rest)—works because it changes the way the body releases hormones, including insulin. The better your body regulates its hormones, the less likely you are to struggle with your weight.

your body a fat-burning machine! And it's not as if you'll look big when you sculpt your muscles. The truth is, women's muscles can get long and lean, but very rarely do women bulk up. Usually, if you see a woman who looks "big" it's really too much fat over muscle.

How to Eat to Lose Weight and Burn Fat

Most people think food is the enemy or contradiction to fat-burning. "If only I could eat less," they think, "Then I could lose weight." But that's not true. Eating is not the opposite of fat-burning, eating *poorly* is the opposite of fat-burning. Eating well is one of the keys to weight loss and fat-burning. Athletes don't starve themselves, they work with nutritionists to design an eating plan that will keep them not only fit and trim, but able to achieve great results with their bodies. This is why you don't want to eat like a dieter, you want to eat like an athlete. Or, at the very least, like a healthy, active person.

To do this, you want to think about only two things:

- Eating whole foods
- Eating proper portions

You'll notice that I didn't tell you to concentrate on what **not** to eat. I believe that giving yourself food restrictions, which is what most diets ask you to do, isn't the way to success. Instead, these two rules will, for the most part, allow you to keep your diet healthy and effective (i.e., they will keep your weight at its proper level and ensure that you get the nutrients you need).

So, let's look at each rule in more detail:

EATING WHOLE FOODS

- Ten strawberries dipped in chocolate vs. two strawberry toaster pastries
- A glass of red wine vs. a diet soda
- A 3-ounce portion of steak with a baked potato vs. a frozen prepared meal

Whole are those foods that can be described as having been grown, farmed, hunted, or slaughtered. Fruits, vegetables, meats, fish, and even wine and chocolate can be included in this group. "Foods" that aren't "whole" would be anything that is manufactured or processed and whose ingredient list includes chemicals or preservatives. A whole food is a potato, as are home-cooked french fries. A non whole-food are french fries made from potato starch, mono- and diglycerides, and potato. Potato in a box is a processed food, not a whole food.

The problem with manufactured and processed foods is that they aren't as nutritious as whole foods. Manufactured french fries, for example, don't have the fiber, vitamins, and minerals that a whole potato has. At the same time, those same french fries have more fat, and it's likely that the fat in those potatoes is of an unhealthy, saturated variety.

Even if you bake the potato and load it with sour cream (a whole food) then you are still eating fewer, more nutritious calories than you will with processed french fries.

I'm going to explore one more example that's a little more extreme: carrot sticks and homemade Ranch dressing vs. pretzels.

The nutritional makeup of two cups of baby carrots with two tablespoons of homemade ranch dressing (using a combination of mayonnaise and buttermilk) would look like this: 75 calories for the carrots and 75 calories for the dressing. The carrots provide almost four grams of fiber; a huge amount of vitamin A; respectable amounts of vitamin C, folate, and other B vitamins; and a nice supply of minerals, such as zinc and calcium. The mayonnaise is high in calories and fat, but added to the carrots, the whole snack is still only about 150 calories and fairly nutritious, not to mention filling.

The pretzels, on the other hand, have the same amount of calories, a fourth of the fiber, and only 1% of most of the nutrients you need throughout the day (they do have a nice amount of folate, but only because the flour has been enriched, and it's still far less than the carrots). And, let's face it, one cup of pretzels isn't that filling.

My point is that even though you've had fat with your carrots, you've still gotten a far better nutritional boost than you did with the pretzels. And, of course, you could always dip your carrots in hummus or nonfat yogurt, which would be even healthier (higher protein, less fat).

You can do this little experiment with any of your favorite "bad" foods (once again, "bad" is anything processed or manufactured). Try to find a whole food alternative (steak vs. bologna, salmon vs. fish sticks, grapes vs. popsicles) and see which food has more vitamins, minerals, and fiber but fewer calories and unhealthy fats—those are the marks of whole foods vs. processed foods.

EATING PROPER PROPORTIONS

The human body needs a specific number of calories to run properly and accomplish with energy and joy the activities it participates in, whether it's working a desk job, running down the beach, playing a game of tag with your kids, or learning a new skill. Calorie is another word for energy and each body requires a certain number of calories to manage its energy.

Most of us in the Western world have an overabundance of food choices and those food choices are often delicious, but they aren't nutritious. And if you eat too much processed food, you'll still be hungry for something nutritious. That's just one reason why you can eat a bag of chips and still be hungry and yet have a bowl of soup or broccoli and feel full.

⊙ GOOD FAT VS. BAD FAT

I've made a few mentions about good fats, bad fats, and saturated fats, so I want to explain what a fat is, what makes it healthy (good) or not healthy (bad), and how fats can be used in your two eating rules (whole foods and portion control).

It's true that, for many years, nutritionists believed that cutting down fat was the secret to good heart health, but now they know that there are (for lack of better terms) good fats and bad fats.

Good fats are monounsaturated and come in the form of fish, avocado, and nuts. Bad fats are saturated and are usually found in meats and dairy products. This doesn't mean you shouldn't eat meat, but it does mean you should choose leaner cuts of meat and low-fat dairy products.

Finally, there is one fat that is the worst. It's partially hydrogenated fat and is only found in processed food (it's not a natural part of food). This is a fat that has been chemically altered to remain shelf-stable (in other words, it keeps your toaster pastries "fresh"). If you see it on the label (you are reading nutrition labels, right?) don't buy it.

The other reason healthy foods fill you up is because of their nutrients. Many healthy foods, especially fruits and vegetables, have lots of water and fiber. These fill up your stomach but aren't high in calories.

Your stomach is only about the size of your two fists put together (make two fists then the place your fingers of each hand against each other). Pretty small, huh? So, when you're planning your meals (and you should be planning them) think about which foods will fill you up with nutrients in your limited amount of space. You'll soon see that a two-fisted meal of a lean protein surrounded by fresh vegetables and a whole grain is the best way to go.

Then, when it's time for dessert, try to have just a few bites (that's really enough) to satisfy your psychological need. Your belly will be full enough from your actual meal to not have room for a big piece of cake.

Putting it All Together

If you eat whole foods, you are less likely to overeat either portions or calories. If you watch your portions, you are less likely to overeat calories and, in turn, to choose unhealthy foods (because whole foods are both bigger in volume and have fewer calories).

It is true that many people need to watch their fat and sugar intake, but by choosing whole foods and watching your portions, you are less likely to eat high-fat and high-sugar foods.

The whole system is really just a circle—one healthy step leads to another—and you can't go wrong if you stay on track.

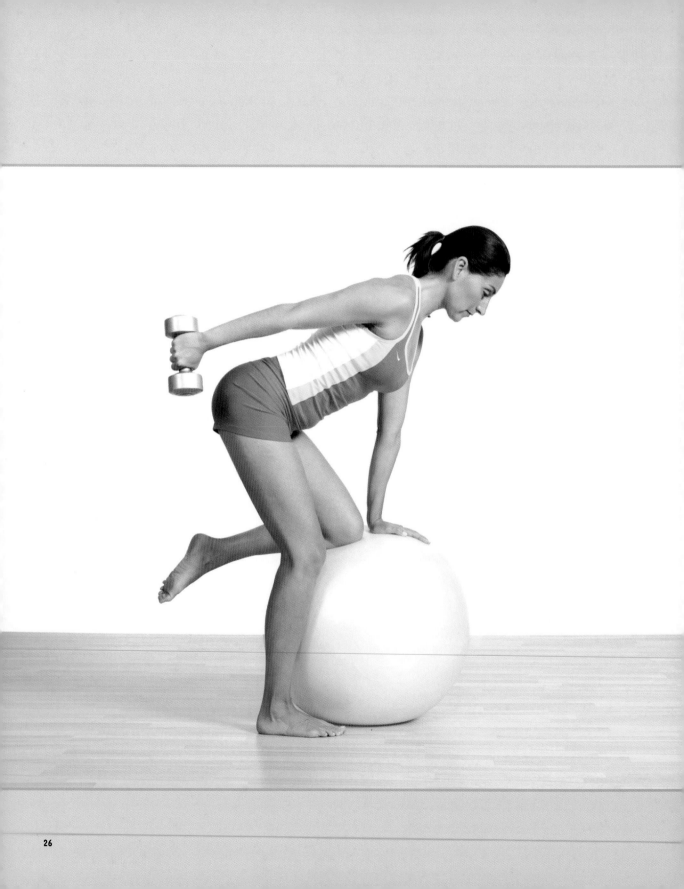

How to Do
These Workouts

his book is a replica (as well as a more extensive spin-off) of my most popular and versatile class: "Work Out on the Ball." This class is an interval program that utilizes the ball for cardio, strength, coordination, balance, and flexibility and everything we do involves the ball—we never put it aside.

We begin the class with a five-minute cardio warm-up to get the body warm and to allow the muscles to loosen up. Then we do a few stretches.

Next, we move into some lower body strengthening work followed by upper body work. We go back to cardio work with more dance-flavored moves—and the ball could be at chest-level, above our heads, or moving around our bodies. Then we go back to the strength-training moves—sometimes using the ball as a resistance tool and sometimes using it to balance. We sit on the ball, dance with it, stand against it, and lie on and over it with every part of our body. We use weights, too, which really help us strengthen our muscles.

We challenge the core muscles throughout the class with side-to-side moves, forward-and-back moves, and up-and-down moves. Alternating in all of these directions not only helps you burn calories, but it adds a balance to your workouts that helps your body develop long, lean muscles equally—you won't overtrain one set of muscles or develop your strength in only one direction, which is common with traditional weightlifting.

What You Need for These Workouts

A BALL

What size ball should you get? Here are some rough sizing guidelines: If you are 4'11" to 5'4" get a 55cm ball. If you are 5'5" to 5'11" get 65cm. If you are 6' or taller get 75cm.

Sizes based upon height are approximate. If you are near a division (for instance, you stand between 5'2" and 5'5" tall) you could opt to go either way. Consider your other body characteristics (such as weight) and how you plan to use the ball.

Filling the ball with air is easily accomplished. The simplest solution is to buy a FitBall hand pump along with your ball (this pump is optional with any of the balls). It makes quick work of inflating. When your ball arrives, here's what you do: remove the plug from the ball, fill the ball with air, then replace the plug.

If you prefer, you can visit your local car or tire repair shop and see if you can use their compressed air machines to blow up the ball.

Wash your exercise ball with a soft cloth and warm, soapy water if it gets dirty.

MUSIC

To make the workout more fun and energetic, I recommend lots of your favorite dance music. While I'm partial to J.Lo and Ricky Martin, you could do these moves to anything with a beat.

I usually play high energy Latin music during class. Many of my steps follow those fast rhythms, which is why they are called Mambo, Cha-Cha, and other dance-inspired names. However, I recommend that you use the music that most inspires you and gets you moving. I love Ricky Martin and Jennifer Lopez, but if rock and roll gets you up, then by all means, use that for your class. You might find that you want to make your own workout CD or podcast so that you can have slower tempo music playing while you lift weights or do your abdominal exercises and have bouncier music on during the cardio segments.

MY MUSIC

These are the CDs I keep in rotation for my class. You can see that we go from high-energy (Ricky Martin and The Gipsy Kings) to the calm and cool (The Buddha Bar collection).

- Cafe Zinho Afternoons — *Frequent Flyer Rio de Janeiro*
- Buddha Bar VII — *Sunangi*
- Buddha Bar VII — *Sarod*
- Buddha Bar VI — *Dinner*
- Time for Peace — *The World Peace 2000*

- Mantra Girl — *Truth*
- Ricky Martin — *Sound Loaded, Ricky Martin*
- Yoga Zone — *Music for Yoga Practice*
- DJ Nia — *Global Unity*
- The Gipsy Kings — *Compass*
- Madonna — *Ray of Light, Immaculate Collection, Confessions on a Dance Floor*
- Jennifer Lopez — *Let's Get Loud, This is Me...Then, J.Lo, The Reel Me, Rebirth*
- Christina Aguilera — *Christina Aguilera*

DUMBBELLS

You will also need dumbbells. I used 5 pound weights during the photo shoot for this book, but for some exercises (specifically those for biceps and shoulders), you might want to try slightly lighter weights. Eventually, you should be able to work yourself up to 5 pounds.

For larger muscle exercises (such as those for the legs and back) you can probably use heavier weights, such as 8 or 10 pound dumbbells. But this is up to you. Some people don't like the hassle of switching weights during a workout. Other people don't mind having two sets next to them as they work out.

LAST BUT NOT LEAST

Finally, you will also need a mat if you don't want to lie on the floor. Also, we do our workouts without shoes, but if you find wearing sneakers more comfortable, by all means, feel free to lace them up.

The Cardio Moves

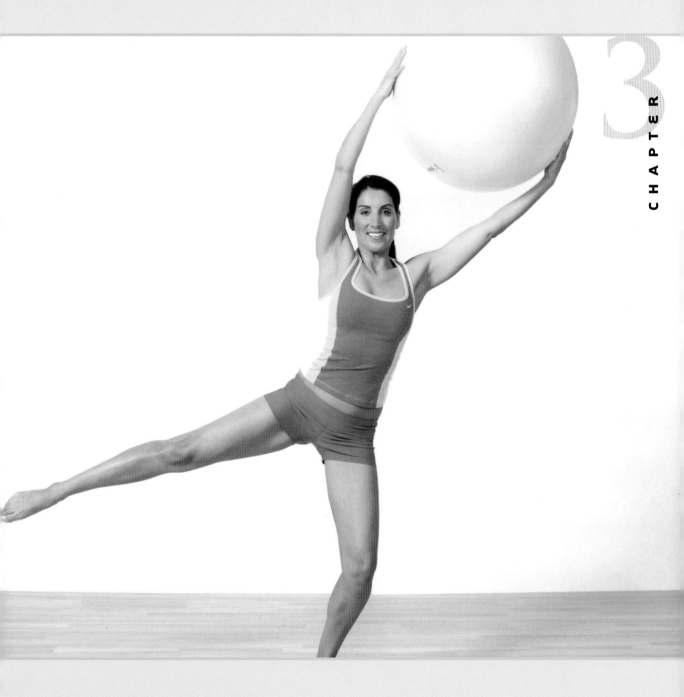

CHAPTER 3

1

Balance Knee
Stretch Front

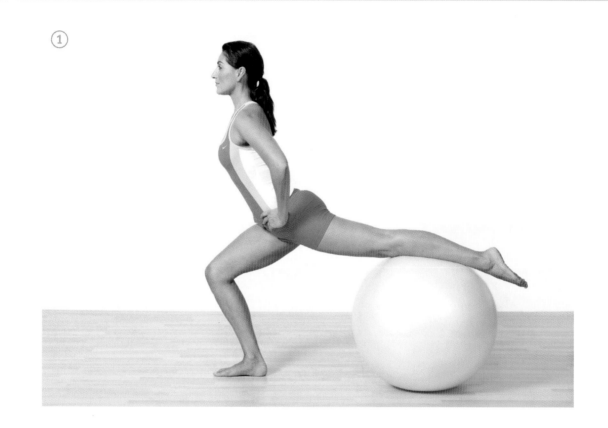

(1) Stand with the ball behind you. Put the top of your right foot on the ball. Hold for 20 seconds.

(2) Roll the ball back and forth, keeping your front knee straight then bending into a one leg squat.

Switch sides. Repeat another set on each side.

Balancing doesn't burn a lot of calories, but it does add an important element to the way a body looks. When you are able to balance, it is likely that your stabilizing muscles are strong. The stabilizing muscles are small and deep and can only be strengthened by actual balancing. You can tell when someone has strong stabilizing muscles because they have good posture and walk steadily and strongly.

Cha-Cha with Mambo

2

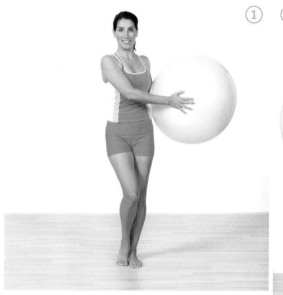 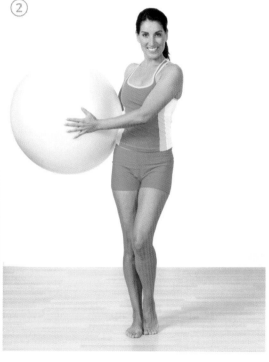

① ②

① Stand with your feet close together, holding the ball at chest level. Be sure your shoulders are relaxed and your torso is long, abs gently contracted.

② Step forward a little bit with your right foot, shifting your weight to that foot. Then quickly return your weight to your left foot, then back to your right foot. Now, step forward with the left foot, shifting your weight to that foot. Then quickly return your weight to your right foot, then back to your left foot.

Dancers have great legs for a number of reasons. First, they burn a lot of calories moving around so much. Second, they use their legs in all ways and in all directions—in strength moves and in lengthening moves. This combination of contraction and relaxation builds muscle and burns fat, which sculpts those muscles into an attractive shape. If you ever have five minutes or an hour, turn on some of your favorite music and dance—it's really one of the best exercises you can do.

3 Cross Step Walk Front with Ball Raise

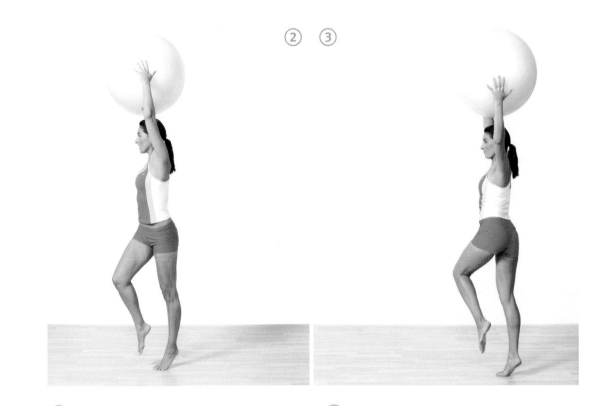

② ③

① Stand with your right foot one step behind your left leg and thighs so close they almost touch (this should look like a sexy model walk) as you hold the ball in front of your chest.

Intensity burns fat. Once you have this move down, you can increase the intensity by moving the body in a "larger" way. That means, stretch your arms longer and bring your knees up higher as you move.

② As you step forward with your right foot, come on to your toes and lift the ball over your head without scrunching up your shoulders. As you take the step, twist your hips toward the left to feel a little strengthening in your right hip and right oblique muscle.

③ Now repeat this with the left foot, twisting your hips to the right. Walk 4-8 steps forward, then walk back. Repeat four times or just about 1 minute.

Double Side Step with Ball Reach Side

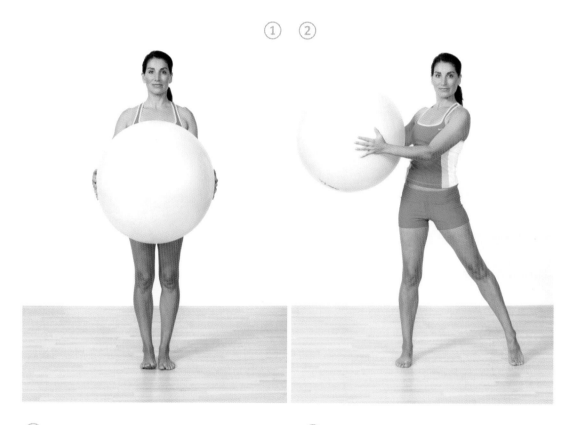

① Stand with feet together, ball in front of your lower torso, shoulders relaxed, body long.

② Step to the right with your right foot, then bring your left foot to your right. Do this once more. As you do this, bring your arms and the ball up to your right side, feeling an elongation and curve in your side. Repeat, starting with your left foot.

Do this in each direction for a full minute.

5

Double Side Step with Ball Twist and Reach

③

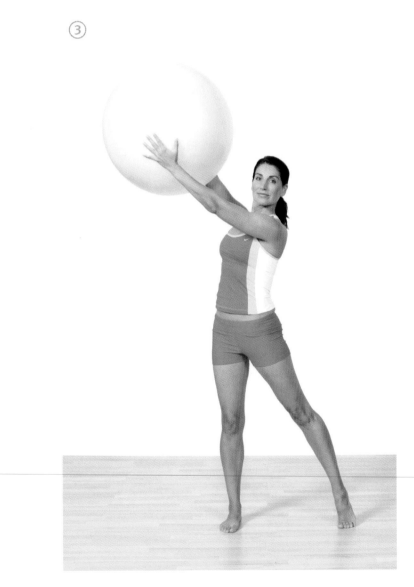

① Stand with your feet hip-width apart, holding the ball just in front of your torso.

② With your right foot, step to the right, bring your left foot in, then step again to the right with your right foot, bring your left foot in. As you step, begin to reach to the right and up with the ball, so that you're twisting to the right.

③ On your final step, the ball should be up and your torso should be turned to the right.

Do this in each direction for a full minute.

Grapevine with Ball Overhead Circles

6

① Stand with your feet together. Lift the ball over your head and hold it there throughout these steps, just to begin.

② Step out to the right with your right foot. Bring your left foot behind your right and then step out to the right with your right foot.

③ As you do this, hold the ball over your head and make a circle in the air, allowing your torso to twist as you move.

Do this 8 times in each direction and go straight into the next move.

③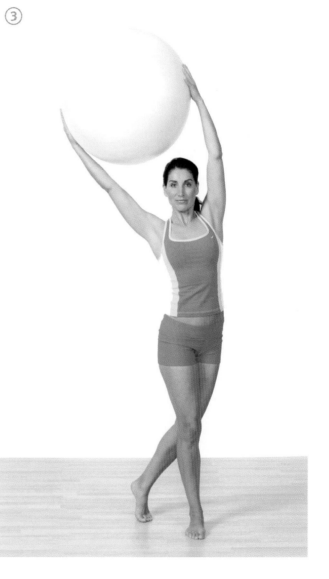

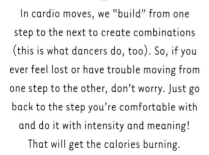

In cardio moves, we "build" from one step to the next to create combinations (this is what dancers do, too). So, if you ever feel lost or have trouble moving from one step to the other, don't worry. Just go back to the step you're comfortable with and do it with intensity and meaning! That will get the calories burning.

7 Kneeling Over Ball: Lean Away with Elbows

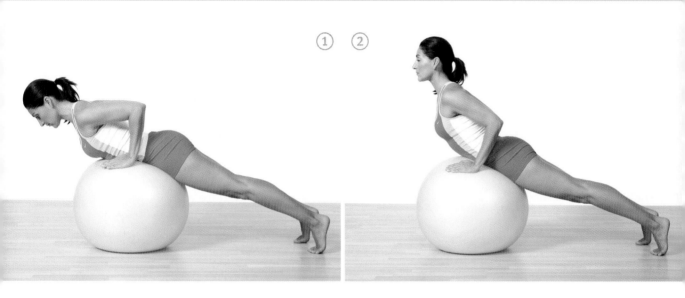

① ②

① With the ball on the floor, put your hands on the top, feet on the floor, body at an angle from the crown of your head to your feet. Make sure your shoulders are away from your ears and your back is long and straight, elbows bent by your sides. Exhale all of your breath.

② Then, on an inhale, lift your chest up to make a long, natural arch in your back. Don't scrunch your shoulders or compress your lower spine by going too high. Instead, feel your body nice and long in an elegant curve.

Hold this for 5 breath cycles (inhale and exhale is one cycle). Then come down. Repeat as many times as you like, focusing on the length of your spine each time.

This move resembles the Cobra from yoga. So take the time to breathe through this pose and relax. It's a wonderful way to stretch your spine and open your chest.

Lay Over Ball:
The Double Leg Lift

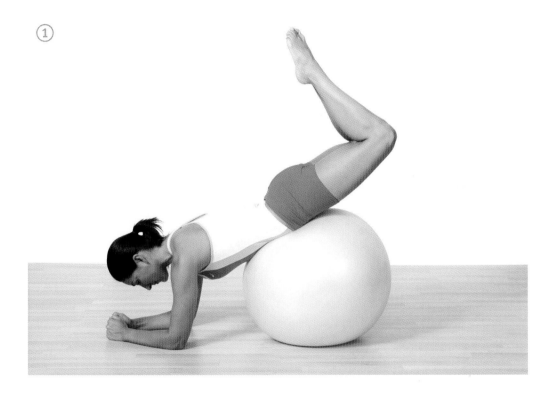

(1) With the ball on the floor, lie over the top. Put your forearms on the floor, hands together, and roll forward so that your legs are at an angle. Bend your knees and point your toes. Keep your neck long and your back straight.

(2) Keeping your legs together, lift your legs up from the ball. This is a very small movement and you'll feel it in your butt. Don't let your back move as you do this, the movement should come from your hips.

Eat more fiber. Like water, fiber can fill you up. It helps your body maintain stable blood sugar levels. Good sources of fiber include brown rice, whole grains, and beans.

9 Lay Over Ball: Leg Lift Circle

① ②

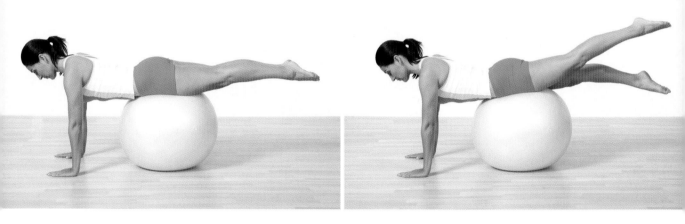

① With the ball on the floor, lie with your belly, hips, and thighs on the ball. Your hands are on the floor in front of the ball, legs out straight, toes pointed. Keep your back in a neutral position, neck long, abs contracted.

If you're going out and feel bloated or just blah, try doing one of my five-minute workouts. You'll start to flush your body out and the energy you'll get from moving vigorously will help improve your mood too.

② Lift your left leg and begin to move it in a small circle, first down, then to the left, then up, then back down. Take your time to stabilize your hips so that you don't allow momentum to take over. Do not move any other part of your body. Your leg should move from your hip, so it won't be able to move in a big circle.

Do this 8 times, then repeat with the other leg.

Lay Chest Over Ball: Back Extension

10

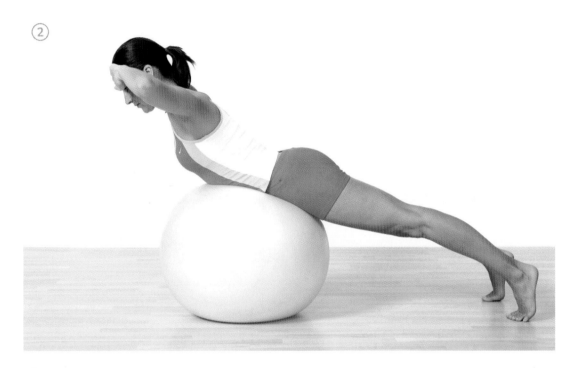

① With the ball on the floor, lie with your hips at the top, your upper body folding forward with your abs contracted. Put the back of your hands against your forehead, fingertips touching, and keep your neck long, shoulders relaxed.

② Keeping your torso long, lift your upper body away from the ball and up, but don't come up past a straight-backed position. In other words, don't overarch your lower back.

Come back to the start position.

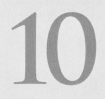

This exercise strengthens your lower back and it's really good if you sit at a desk or in a car for long periods of time. If you have lower back pain, you might try just lying over the back with your lower back at the top. Let your hips, legs, and upper body hang over the ball (let the ball support you completely). Your upper and lower body will act as weights and stretch your lower back. (You can reverse this—lie on your back—to stretch out your abs and chest too.)

11 Lay Chest Over Ball: Back and Arm Extension

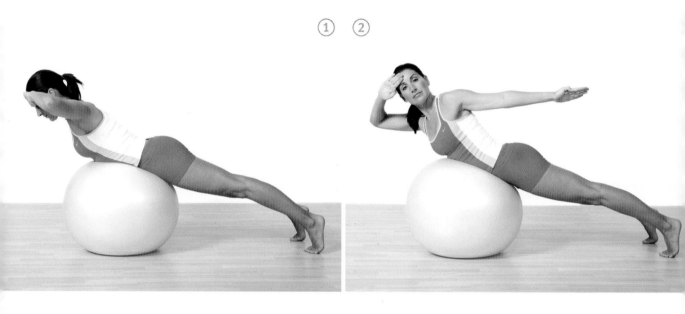

① ②

① With the ball on the floor, lie with your belly on the top, your body in a long, straight line from your head to your toes. Put the back of your hands against your forehead, fingertips touching, and keep your neck long, shoulders relaxed.

② Keeping your torso long, lift your upper body away from the ball and up, but don't overarch your back. As you get to the top of the position, extend your arm and turn to the left slightly. Don't twist, just turn.

Come back to the start position and repeat to the other side.

Mambo with Ball Twist

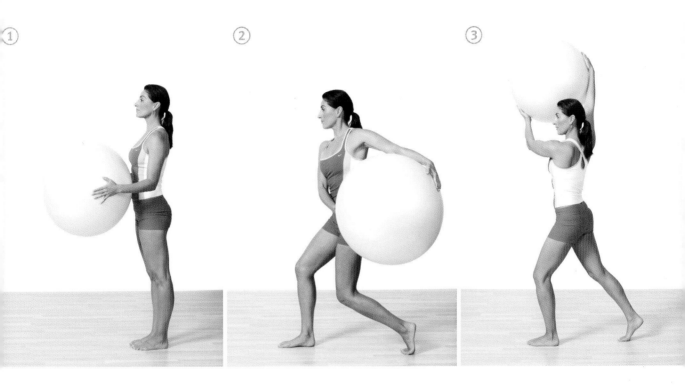

① Turn to the side and stand with the ball in front of your torso.

② Step forward with your right foot and put all your weight onto your right leg. As you do this, bring the ball down to your left side by your hips so that your torso twists a little bit in opposition.

③ On your next step, bring your right leg to the back while you bring the ball up to the right, over your head. This changes the direction of your torso twist.

Make sure you eat after your workout. It's best to have something high in protein (such as a hard-boiled egg, a slice of hard cheese, or some turkey) and some complex carbs (such as an apple, raisins, or berries). This will help restore your glucose levels so you don't get tired and the protein will both build muscle and keep your blood sugar levels up longer than if you just ate the carbs.

13 March in Place with Ball Held at Chest Level

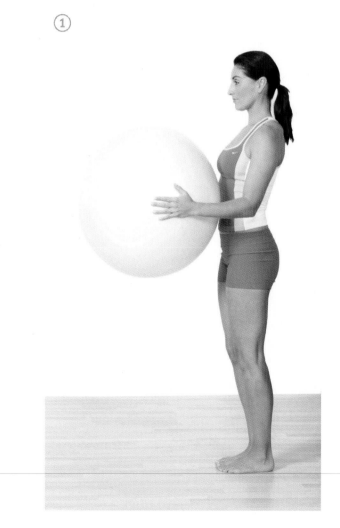

①

① Stand with your feet together, shoulders away from your ears, ball in your hands. Step high, bending your knees. As you do this, hold the ball in front of you. Try to keep your chest high.

Do this 16 times (8 times with each foot).

Marching or walking in place is a great exercise to do if you're watching TV. Believe it or not, if you walk in place for a half hour, you will have walked the equivalent of somewhere between $1^1/_2$ to 2 miles (depending on your stride length and how fast you are going). So don't dismiss this as a throw-away exercise. You can burn 150 calories and really make a difference in your body!

March in Place with Ball Overhead Reaches

14

(1) Stand with your feet together, shoulders away from your ears, ball in your hands.

(2) Step high, bending your knees. As you do this, move the ball up and down over your head. This will bring you heart rate up even more.

Do this 16 times (8 times with each foot).

(2)

Are you watching your TV and marching in place? Bring the ball into your workout. You can raise it up and over your head, move it around your body as you march, or use it in place to do some exercises while the commercials are on. Check out the five-minute routines starting on page 165. Those are great for commercial breaks.

15 March in Place with Ball Twist

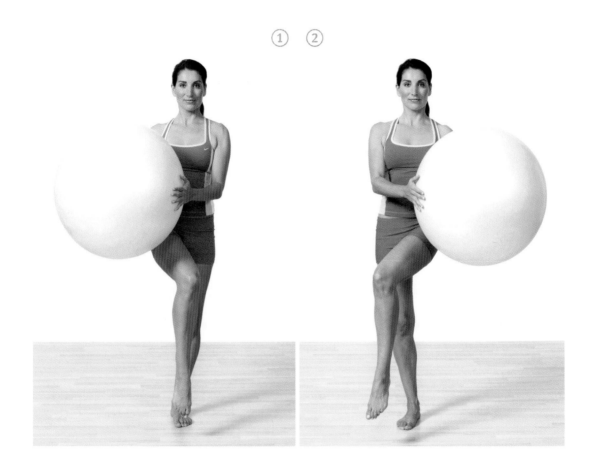

① ②

① Stand with feet together, ball in front of your torso.

② March in place, turning slightly to the side with each step. You should feel a slight stretch and strengthening in your side abdominal muscles (the obliques). Keep your shoulders relaxed and your torso long.

Do this 16 times (8 times on each foot).

Seated Pliés with Ball between Legs and Squeeze

16

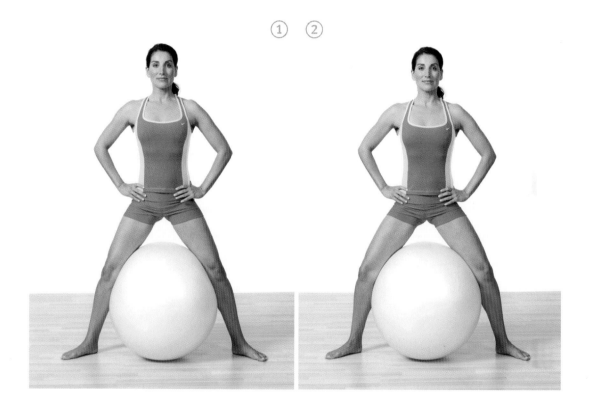

(1)   Stand with the ball between your legs and resting on the floor. Place hands on hips. Bend into a plié, using the ball as a guide for your thighs.

(2)   Touch the ball with your thighs (but do not sit on it), pressing them back against the ball for a second, then come back up. Come down on a count of two, come up on a count of two.

Do this 16 times.

The inner thighs are just one of those areas women find difficult to tone. This exercise will help a lot. Here's another one you can do when you're watching TV or just lying in bed: lie on your back, legs up in the air. Now, cross your lower legs and feet back and forth across each other. You can do this fairly rapidly. Keep your legs long and straight. You can do this with pointed toes or flexed feet and you should feel it in your inner thighs.

17

Side Step "Step Touch" with Ball Twist

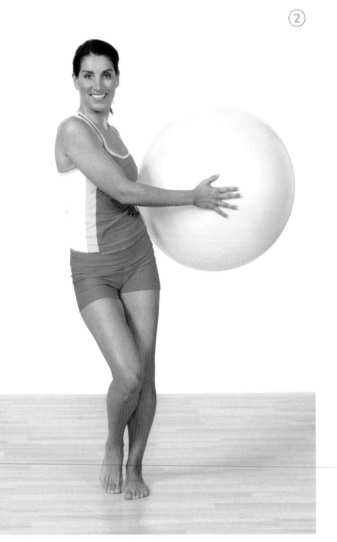

① Stand with feet together, ball in your hands.

② Step to the right with your right foot, then bring your left foot to touch your right foot. As you do this, twist to the right with the ball and your upper body.

Do the same thing to the other side. If you can, try to jump from side to side or bring your knees up as you move to raise your heart rate.

Do this 16 times (8 times on each side).

Once you're used to these moves, feel free to increase the intensity by doing longer sequences or changing them up as you want to. Part of the joy of using the ball is being creative and challenging yourself.

Sideways Mambo with Ball Raises

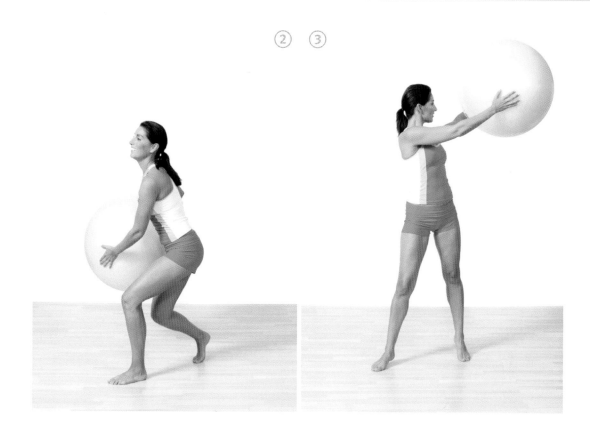

① Stand at a slight angle with the ball in front of you, feet close together. Step forward with your right foot, then quickly shift your weight back to your left foot. Then go back to your right foot quickly.

② As you do this, bring the ball down to your knee during the first step.

③ Then bring it up over your shoulder on the final step back. You should move the ball and your torso smoothly so that it looks as if you're dancing the mambo.

Do this 16 times on each leg.

19 Standing Pliés with Ball Side Twist

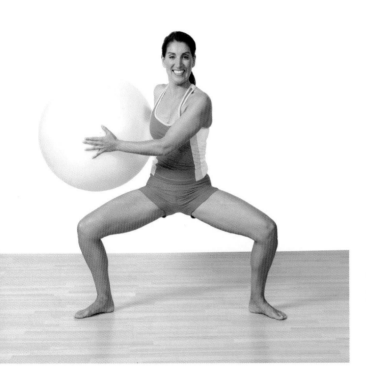

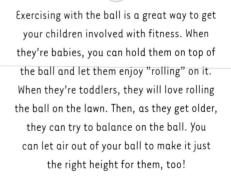

① Stand with your feet further than hip-width apart, toes turned out, but hips under your shoulders (i.e., your butt isn't sticking out and your pelvis isn't tucked forward). Bend your knees into a plié, making sure that if you look down, you can see your toes in front of your knee.

② As you bend, move the ball to your right and twist your torso. Be sure to keep your hips steady. The move is a twist for your core abdominals, the obliques, and transverse abdominus.

Come back to center, then go to the left. Repeat 8 times on each side.

Exercising with the ball is a great way to get your children involved with fitness. When they're babies, you can hold them on top of the ball and let them enjoy "rolling" on it. When they're toddlers, they will love rolling the ball on the lawn. Then, as they get older, they can try to balance on the ball. You can let air out of your ball to make it just the right height for them, too!

Standing Side Lunges with Low Ball Reach

20

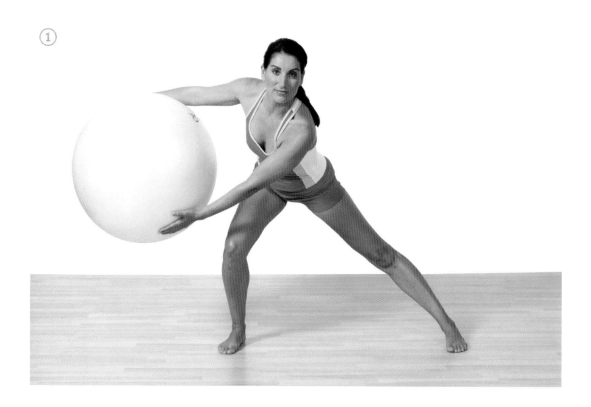

① Stand with your feet together, ball in front of your torso. Step out to the right side with your right foot, going into a side lunge. Bring the ball down toward your right side.

② Be sure your right knee doesn't go past your right toes. Come back to center, then go to the left. This is a tough move to do, so don't be surprised if you do this more slowly than other moves.

Do this 16 times (8 times on each side).

Your heart health is measured not by how hard it can work, but by how fast and how fully it can recover from working hard. If you find it difficult to catch your breath after the cardio portion of a workout or if your heart is still beating fast about ten minutes after you body slows down, go see a doctor and tell her about this symptom.

21 Step Touch with Ball Twist

① ②

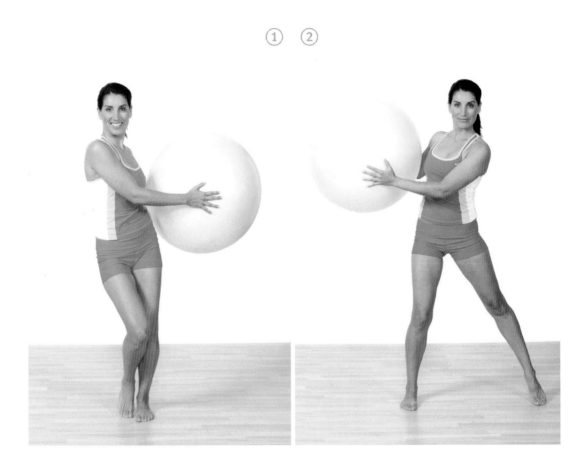

① Stand with your feet together, ball in front of your torso, knees slightly bent. Step to your right with your right foot and bring the ball out to your right side.

② Then step to your left while bringing the ball to your right side.

Do this 16 times (8 on each side).

Tap Side with a Twist and Turn

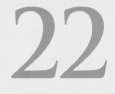

① ②

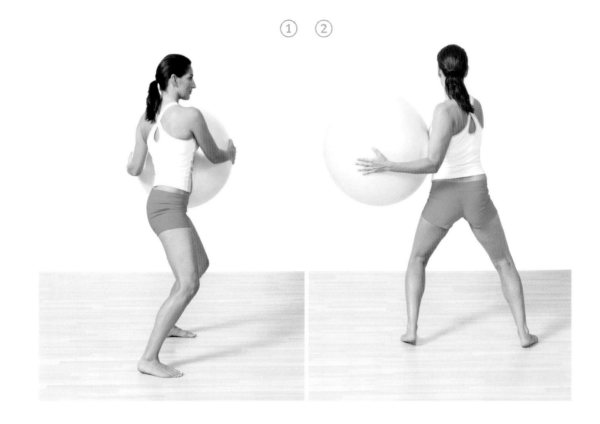

① Stand with your legs further than hip-width apart, ball in front of your torso. Lunge to the right, but don't go down into the lunge. Instead, bend your knee and reach up with the ball as you raise your left leg as high as comfortable, keeping a slight bend in your left knee and feeling the stretch in your hips. Now, start tapping your foot on the floor in a circle around your body to turn.

This move is an almost perfect leg shaper. It strengthens your hamstrings (back of the thighs), quadriceps (front of the thighs), gluteals (butt), and the calves. It works so well because you are putting all of your body weight onto one leg. Research has shown that one-legged squats are the most effective leg and butt shaper you can do.

23 Tap Side with Ball Twist

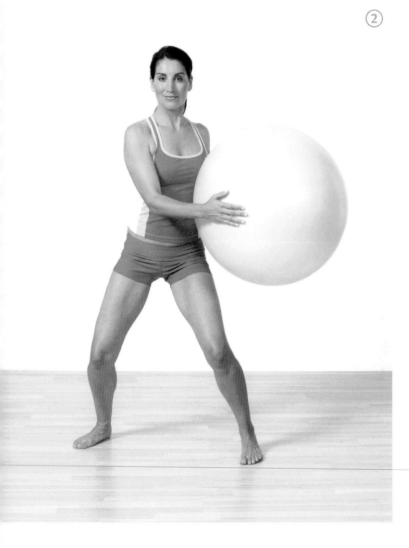

② ① Stand with the ball in front of your torso, feet about shoulder-width apart. Step out widely to the right side with your right foot, making sure to bend your knees, but don't go quite into a plié. This is a fast-tempo move. Keep the weight of your feet light to keep yourself moving quickly.

② As you step to the side, twist your torso to the opposite side of your moving leg. Keep your abs contracted so you feel the move in your oblique muscles. You'll also feel it in your thighs (front and back) and butt.

Repeat this move on the left side.

This is a dance-y move, so just let yourself go and move with it quickly. Don't worry if you're doing it "right." Instead, feel the beat of the music and just move around in a circle.

Traveling Side Chasé with Ball Overhead Circles

24

(1) Stand with your feet together, ball in front of your torso. Do a side skip (step to the right, bring your left foot in, then step to your right again quickly) to your right side while bringing the ball around, up and over your head. The last part of this sideways movement ends with the ball above your head and your left leg out to the side. Come down and do the same thing to the left.

This move is traditionally called a chasé in dance and is like a quick slide with a little jump in between. Repeat 16 times (8 on each side).

(1)

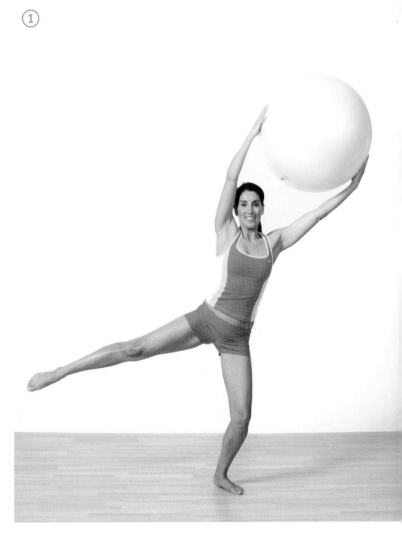

25 Circle Walk with Ball Twist

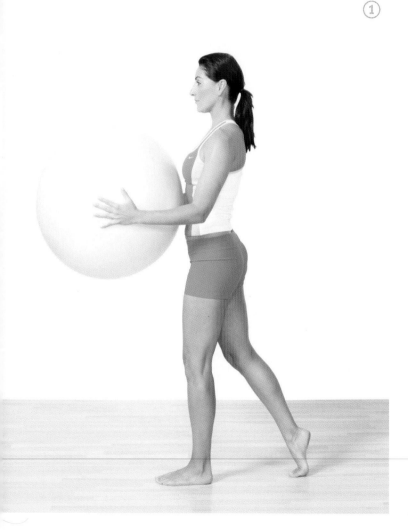

① ① Start with your right foot, and walk in place for four steps. Then turn right and walk around in a circle, making eight steps. Turn the ball up and down as you walk. After completing the circle, walk in place for three steps and finish with a quick tap with your left foot. Lead with the left foot, this time making eight steps in a circle to the left. Finish by walking in place again.

Do this 8 times (4 times in each direction.

Once you're used to this beat and combination, you can increase the intensity by making your walk more exciting. Try skipping, marching, or running your steps.

Walk Front/Back with Ball Overhead Reach

26

(1) Stand with the ball at chest height. Walk forward four counts, raise the ball over your head and back down four times as you move your feet. Next, walk back four counts and raise the ball over your head and back down four times as you walk.

Do this 8 times.

(1)

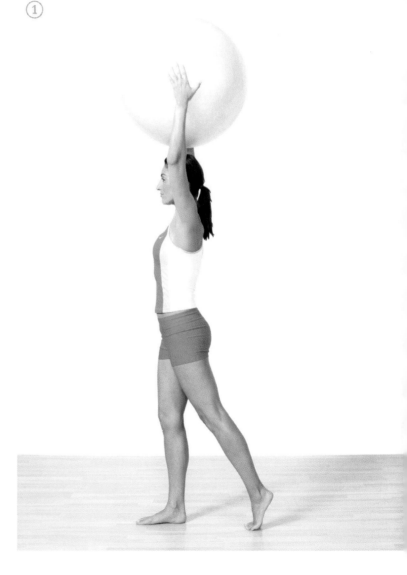

27 Walk in Place with Ball Held at Chest Level

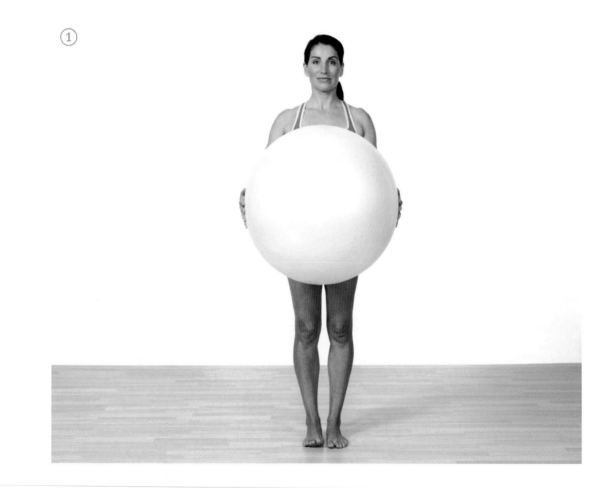

① Stand with your feet close together, holding the ball at chest level, elbows down, shoulders down. Walk in place as you hold the ball. Try to bring your knees up high (this is where your heart rate starts rising).

If you're holding the ball right in front of your body, squeeze it with your hands for an added pectoral (chest) strengthener. The resistance will help build strength in your pecs and give your breasts some lift!

The Strengthening and Toning Moves

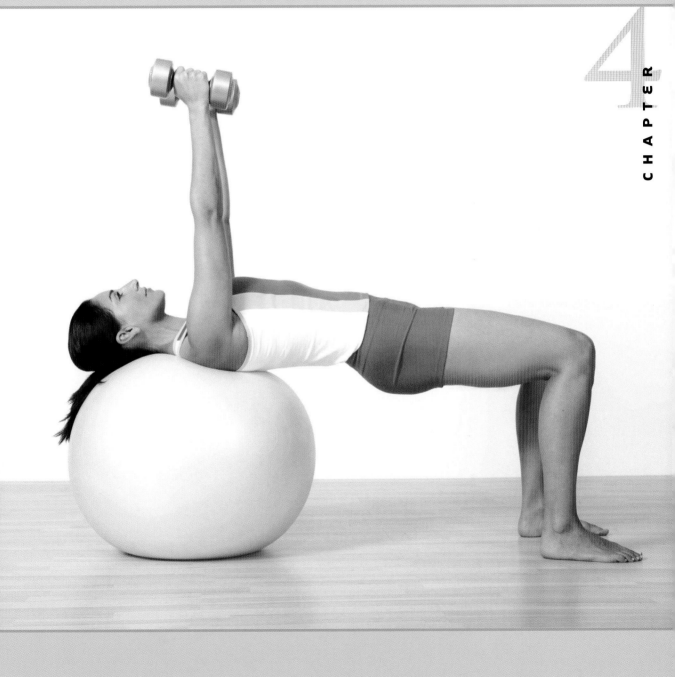

CHAPTER 4

28

Incline Chest Squeeze

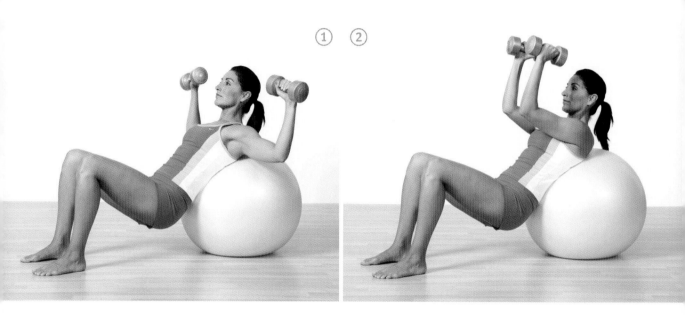

① ②

① With the ball on the floor, lie on the top holding a dumbbell in each hand, and keep your feet on the floor. Now, roll down the ball so your shoulders and back are supported by the ball. Your knees should be bent and your abs and butt can be relaxed, but not sagging. Let the ball support your upper arms. Hold your forearms up with the weight at head height. This is your start position.

② Without raising your shoulders, bring your elbows and forearms together so you feel (and see, if you look down) a squeeze in your chest. You probably

won't be able to bring your elbows to touch, but get them as close together as possible in order to achieve the "squeeze" effect. Return to the start position.

Do this 8 times.

⊚

As women get older, changes in hormone levels can mean changes in their breasts, including size, shape, and health. Exercise has been shown to greatly affect—in a positive way—hormone levels in the body, so as you do this exercise, remember that weightlifting is good not only for your outer health (the way you look) but also your inner health (the way you feel).

Lay Over Ball: Reverse Fly with Dumbbells

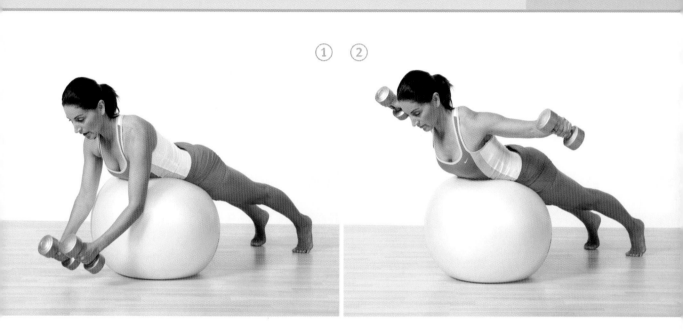

① ②

① With the ball on the floor, lie on top with your belly pressed against it. Your arms and hands should be down with slightly bent elbows, in front of the ball, each holding a dumbbell. Neck long, shoulders relaxed, legs out straight, toes on floor.

② On an exhale and without moving your back, raise your arms out to the sides with slightly bent elbows, coming out only as high as your shoulders. Inhale and bring your arms back to start. You should feel this right in the middle of your back.

30 Kneeling over Ball: Single Arm Row with Dumbbells

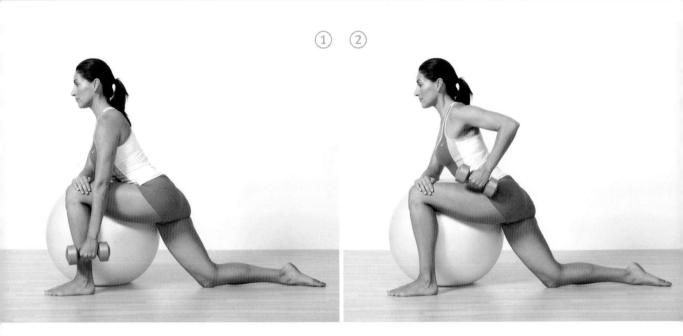

① ②

① With the ball on the floor, go into a lunge with your right leg on the floor and your left leg bent next to the ball. Hold a dumbbell in your left hand and have your right elbow on the ball. The ball should be tucked into your thighs. This will keep your body in alignment as you do the move.

② Look straight ahead as you keep your back at a slight angle. While keeping your elbow close to your body, bend your elbow and bring the weight in to your hip. You should feel this on the sides of your back.

Repeat this move 8-16 times on each side.

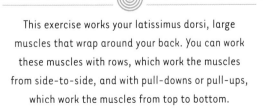

This exercise works your latissimus dorsi, large muscles that wrap around your back. You can work these muscles with rows, which work the muscles from side-to-side, and with pull-downs or pull-ups, which work the muscles from top to bottom.

Kneeling on Ball: Triceps Extension

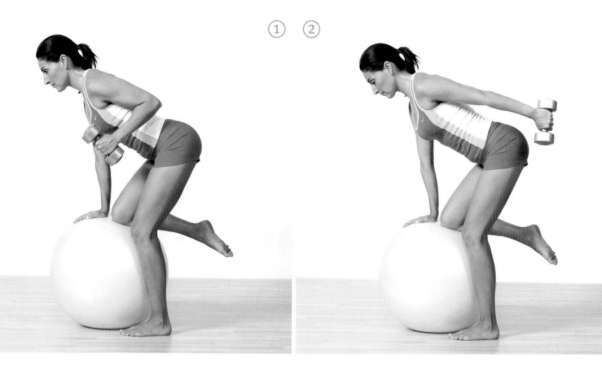

(1) (2)

(1) With the ball on the floor, put your right knee and right hand on top, hold a dumbbell in your left hand, elbow bent, weight just under your shoulder. Keep your back straight, abdominals contracted, and neck straight.

(2) Straighten your elbow but don't come to a locked position. Instead, focus on feeling the contraction in the back of your upper arm.

Switch sides and repeat 8 times on each side.

Triceps respond very well to using heavier dumbbells, so don't be afraid to go up to eight or ten pounds when doing this exercise. If you really want to see a difference in the shape of your upper arms, you'll need to work hard and that means heavier weights.

32

Lay Back Over Ball: Chest Fly with Dumbbells

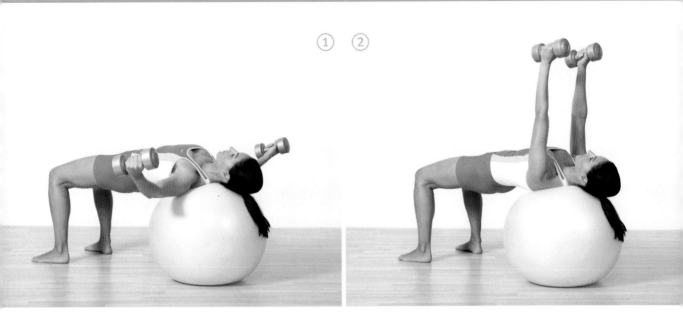

① ②

① With the ball on the floor, put your upper back on top, shoulders at the top, neck and head supported. Your feet should be on the floor, thighs pointed slightly down. Hold a dumbbell in each hand, arms above your head, shoulders relaxed away from your ears.

② Bring your arms out and down to the sides, leading with your elbows. Do not go below chest height. Now, bring your arms back up, squeezing your pectoral muscles together at the top.

Do this 8 times. Rest, then repeat.

The pectoral, or chest, muscle is really three muscles in one. The muscle begins under your breastbone in the center of your chest and then fans out in three directions—to your shoulder, to your side just under your arm, and down to your side just above your waist. If you want to give yourself extra lift and better posture, you can do this exercise in three positions. The one I demonstrate works the mid-pectoral muscle. To work the top part of your chest, roll down on the ball so that your arms meet higher on your chest. To work the bottom, roll back on the ball (in a decline position) so that the lower part of your chest is higher than the rest.

Lay Back Over Ball: Chest Press with Dumbbells

33

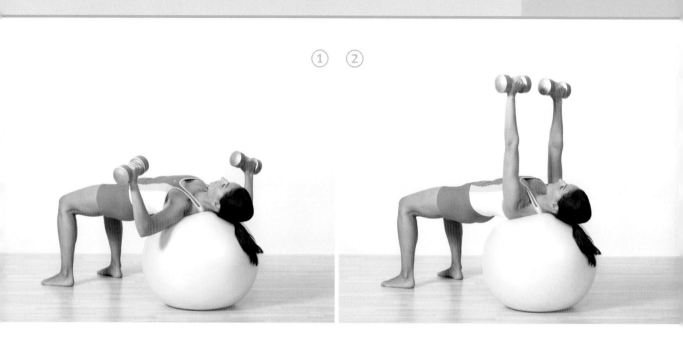

① ②

① With the ball on the floor, lie with your back on the ball, chest at the top, neck and head supported. Hold a dumbbell in each hand and bring your arms out to the sides, elbows bent. Your upper arms are pointed slightly down and your forearms are perpendicular to the floor, shoulders away from the ears.

② Contract your pectoral muscles, then straighten your arms, bringing your hands and the weights together. You should feel and see your chest squeeze together at the top of the move.

Return your arms to the start position. Do this 8 times. Rest, then repeat.

The chest press works a different aspect (or section) of the pectoral muscles—the middle, between your breasts. Most women can use heavier weights with these exercises than just light dumbbells. Try 10 to 15 pounds to see how it feels. You'll notice a real difference in your shape if you use heavier weights. (Remember, weightlifting can't change the size of your breasts, but it can give you some lift.)

34

Lay Back Over Ball: Cross Triceps Extensions with Dumbbells

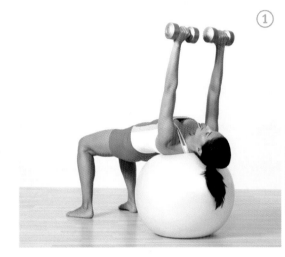

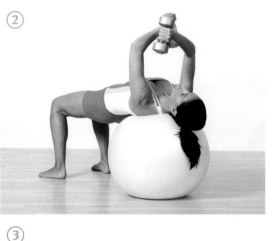

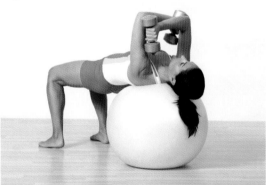

① With the ball on the floor, lie with your neck, shoulders, and upper body on the top of the ball. Your feet are on the floor, knees bent, thighs pointed slightly down. Hold a dumbbell in each hand, arms up high over your head, palms facing away from you.

② Lower both your hands toward the opposite shoulders, keeping the weight facing away from you.

Return to the start. Do this 8 times.

This exercise is an excellent complement to the Triceps Extension because it works a different aspect of the triceps muscle, so you're toning a slightly different part of your upper arm.

Lay Back Over Ball: The Go-Go with Dumbbells

35

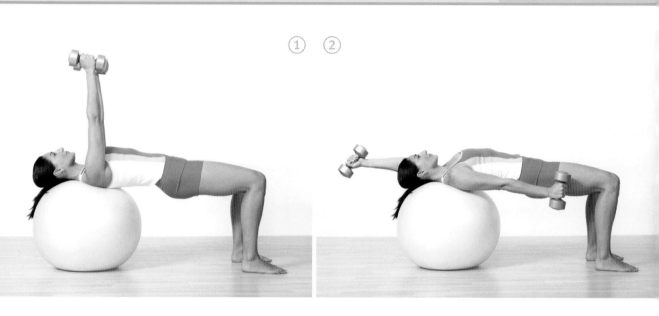

① Sit on the ball, holding a dumbbell in each hand. Roll forward so that your upper back is lying against the ball. Keep your hips up in a tabletop position. Your knees should be just over your ankles. Start with your arms straight up over your head.

② Now, lower your arms and bring your left arm up alongside your ear, pointed slightly down, at the same time you bring your right arm down alongside your thigh.

Switch arm positions. Do this 8 times for each arm.

This is a variation of a Pilates exercise, which uses light weights and a focus on the position of small muscles within the body to bring length and strength to your body.

36 Lay Back Over Ball: Pull Over with Dumbbells

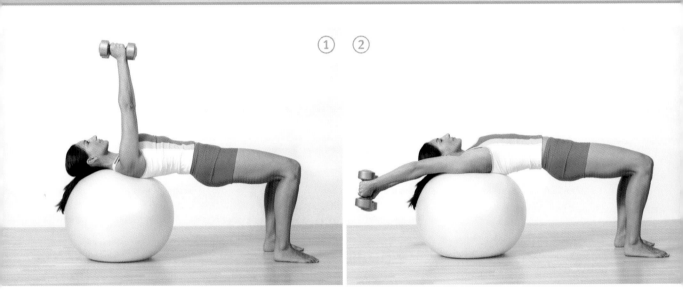

① ②

① Sit on the ball with a dumbbell in each hand. Step your feet out and roll down the ball so that you end with the ball under your shoulders and upper back. Your torso and legs should be in a tabletop position, knees parallel to each other, thighs pointed slightly down, shins perpendicular to the floor. Raise your arms straight over your head, hands facing each other. Keep your neck and shoulders relaxed.

② Lower your arms behind your head without scrunching up your shoulders.

You should feel a stretch in your chest. Don't lower your arms past your ears.

Bring your arms to the start position. Do this 8 times. Rest, then repeat.

Drink plenty of water. Being hydrated plays a critical role in your body's ability to burn fat and achieve total fitness. By the time you're thirsty, you're already dehydrated; so keep a water bottle by your side throughout the day.

Lay Over Ball: Double Leg Hamstring Curl with Dumbbell

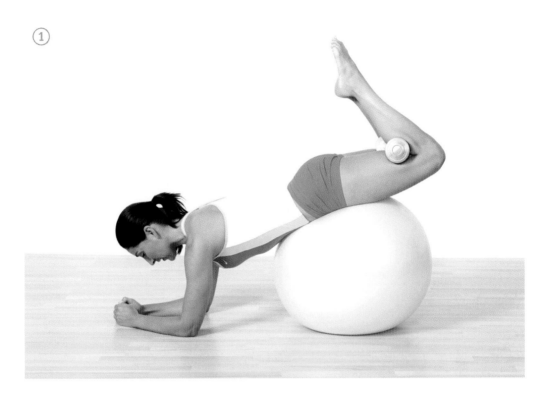

① Lie with your abdominals over the ball and put a dumbbell against the backs of both knees. Roll forward on the ball and rest your forearms on the floor, hands clasped, elbows out.

② Lift your legs from the hips, using your gluteal muscles.

Do this 8 times. Rest, then repeat.

38 Lay Over Ball: Flutter Kick

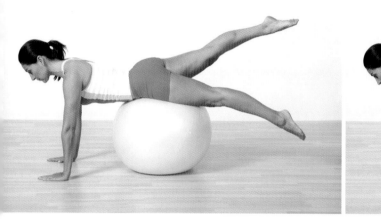

① ②

① With the ball on the floor, lie on the top with your belly and hips centered. Put your hands on the floor in front of the ball and hold your legs out straight, toes pointed. Keep your neck long and your abs contracted.

② Moving just from your hips, begin to move your left and right legs in kicks in opposition. Don't let your hips move; instead, feel the muscles in your butt, inner thighs, and hamstrings contract as you move your legs.

Do this 8 times. Rest, then repeat.

When you do this exercise, you should really focus on making the movement small even though that might seem counter-intuitive. During a cardio program, we know that moving bigger means burning more calories, but when you're doing a strength move, small motions mean more control and more muscle contraction.

Lay Over Ball: Hamstring Curl with Dumbbell

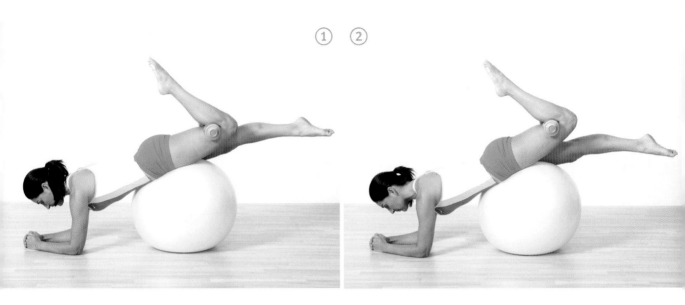

(1) Lie with your abdominals over the ball, arms and legs long, put a dumbbell in one bent knee and keep the other leg long. Roll forward, bringing your forearms to the floor in front of the ball. Clasp your hands together and make a triangle with your arms.

(2) Lift the bent knee, feeling the squeeze in your butt. You'll only go up a few inches. Return to the start position. Be sure you don't move the rest of your body, especially your lower back.

Do this 8 times. Rest, then repeat.

Some people find it really difficult to keep the dumbbell in their knee, but this is effective even without the extra weight, so if you find it too hard to use the extra pounds, just skip them. Or, better yet, use ankle weights that you can Velcro on.

40

Lay Chest Over Ball:
Lat Pull with Leg Extension

① ②

① With the ball on the floor, lie with your chest on top, right hand resting on the floor, left arm extended at an angle toward the floor holding a dumbbell. Your left toe should rest on the floor while your right leg is extended behind you, out straight. This is the start position.

② Now, as if you are starting a lawn mower, bend your left elbow and pull your left arm up. As you do this, extend your right leg higher and really feel the contraction in the muscles below your shoulder blade and in your glute.

(This is a compound move, which means you are strengthening the muscles in more than one body part).

Return to the start position. Do this 8 times. Rest, then repeat.

The start position alone is an exercise for your back. Because you are balancing with your core muscles and extending opposite limbs, you are giving your back a stretch and a strengthening move at once.

Lay Chest Over Ball: Push-Ups

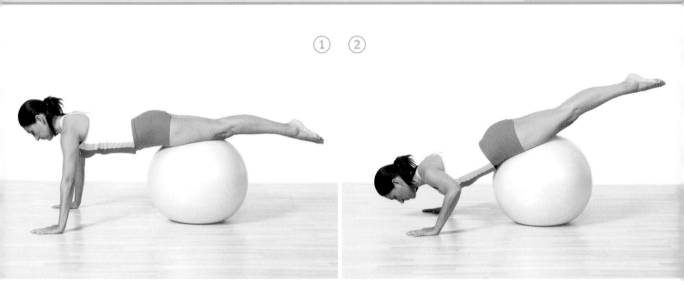

① ②

① With the ball on the floor, put your upper body on the ball, legs out straight, and then roll forward on the ball, so that your thighs rest on the ball and your hands hold your upper body off the floor, body at an angle. Your body should be straight, abs contracted, neck straight, eyes on the floor. This is the start position.

② Bend your elbows and lower your head, neck, chest, and shoulders toward the floor without letting your torso sag or your butt stay up in the air.

Return to the start position. Do this 8 times. Rest, then repeat.

This is a decline push-up, but since the ball is supporting some of your weight, it might not be as difficult for you as a traditional straight-legged push-up. If you do find it difficult, that's good—it means you'll make a lot of progress the more you practice it. Here's a tip: do what you can on the ball, then go down to the floor and do as many bent-legged push-ups as you can to really train your pectoral muscles. Pretty soon you'll work your way to the full count of straight-legged ones.

42 On the Floor: Abdominal Curl with Leg Extension

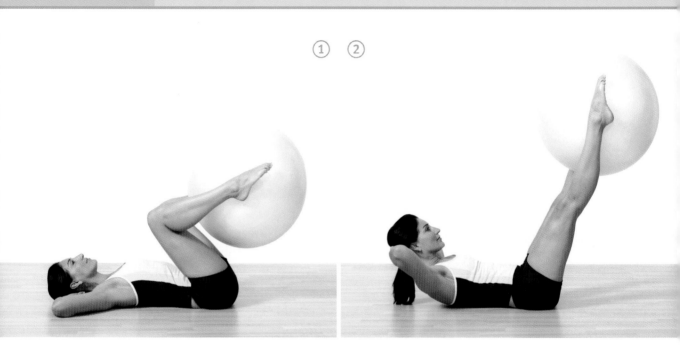

① ②

① Lie on the floor, back gently pressed to the floor, hands behind your head, elbows out. The ball should be between your feet and lower legs, knees bent, toes pointed, abs contracted, hips even on the floor.

② On an exhale, bring your head, neck, and shoulders off the floor as you straighten your legs. Keep your back gently pressed to the floor. You should feel this in your abs.

On an inhale, come down slowly. Do this 8 times. Rest, then repeat.

On the Floor: Crisscross

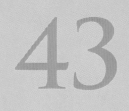

①

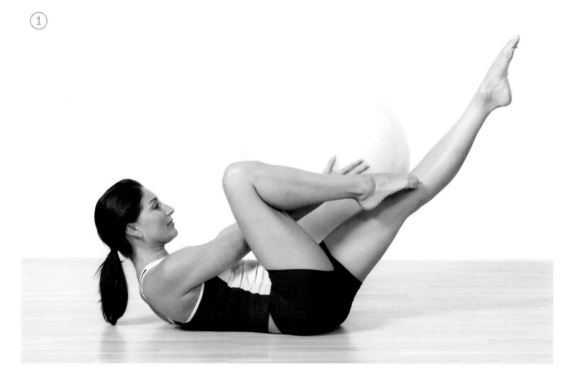

① Lie on your back with the ball in your hands, above your torso. Press your lower back gently onto the floor as you raise your legs to a 45-degree angle from your hips. Keeping your shoulders away from your ears, raise your head, neck, and shoulders off the floor.

② Bend your right knee and bring it in toward your chest. As you do this, twist toward your left slightly, bringing your hand and the ball down toward your left knee.

Continue to switch legs as the ball moves up and over toward the outside leg. Do this 8 times on each side. Rest, then repeat.

44

On the Floor: Double Leg Lift Side with Inner Thigh Squeeze

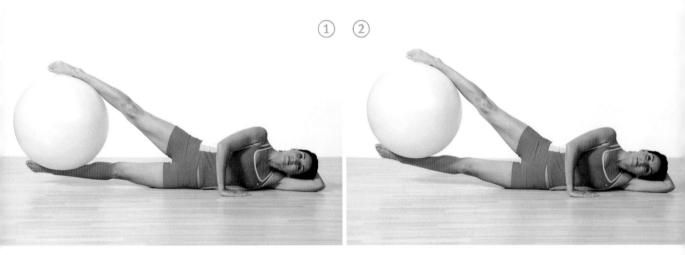

① ②

① Lie with your left side on the floor, arm under head, right hand resting on the floor in front of your chest. Put the ball between your feet, ankles, and shins. Stack your hips, one over the other, so they stay in alignment.

② Raise the ball a few inches above the floor. This is the start position. Raise your legs a few inches more. Be sure the rest of your body feels long and straight. You should feel this on the outside of your right thigh and on the inside of your left thigh.

Do this 8 times on each side. Rest, then repeat.

◎

This exercise strengthens the obliques and outside of your thigh, which aren't easy spots to tone. To make a difference in these parts of your body, you need to focus on small, precise movements.

On the Floor: Hip Rolls with Leg Extension

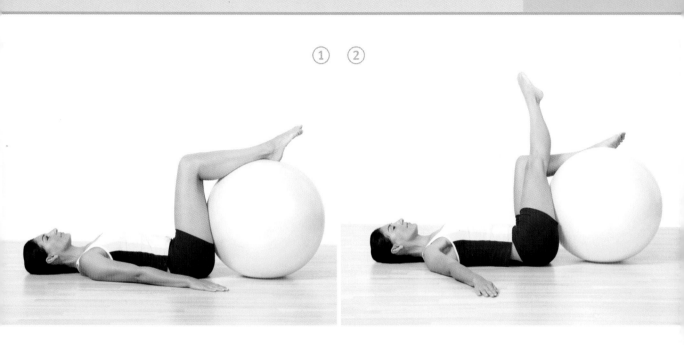

45

(1) Lie on the floor with the ball just in front of your butt, both legs across the ball, arms out from your sides at a slight angle on the floor. Be sure your back is gently against the floor.

(2) On an exhale, tilt your hips toward the left without letting your ribs and upper back lose contact with the floor. Let the ball roll with you, then on the twist, extend the right leg up in the air.

On an inhale, return to the start position. Roll to the other side and extend the left leg. Do this 8 times on each side. Rest, then repeat.

46

On the Floor: Inner Thigh Squeeze with Abdominal Curl

①

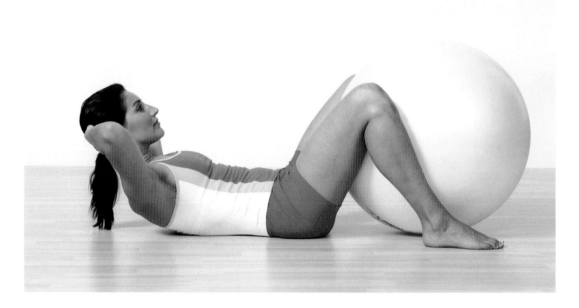

① Lie on the floor with your back flat and your knees bent. The ball should be between your legs. Put your hands behind your head and keep your elbows bent, out to the sides.

② As you raise your head, squeeze your thighs together against the ball. Keep your eyes focused on the wall in front of you, high above your knees, but don't look up to the ceiling. Keep your back pressed gently toward the floor. Come down.

Do this 8 times. Rest, then repeat.

Eat. Your body begins to burn calories when you exercise and if you don't eat, your body holds onto the calories it has stored. This isn't a license to eat saturated fat and sugar. Instead, it means you should eat healthy fats and proteins, complex carbohydrates, fruit, and other whole foods.

On the Floor: Inner Thigh Squeeze with Oblique Arm Reach

47

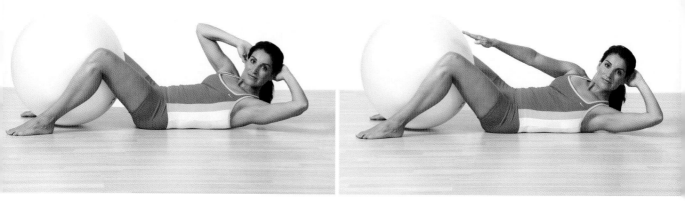

① ② Lift your head, shoulders, neck, and

① Lie on the floor with the your knees bent, feet down, back flat, hands behind your head, elbows bent and out to the sides.

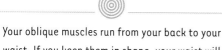

Your oblique muscles run from your back to your waist. If you keep them in shape, your waist will be trimmer and your core will feel stronger.

② Lift your head, shoulders, neck, and upper back up and turn to the left as you squeeze the ball between your legs. Reach your right arm up and over your left knee. Keep your lower back pressed to the floor and your neck long. You shouldn't feel any tension in your body, just a contraction in your oblique muscle (it wraps around your waist). Come back down.

Do this 8 times on each side. Rest, then repeat.

48

On the Floor: Inner Thigh Squeeze with Roll Up

① ②

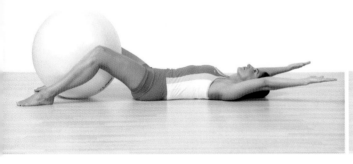

③

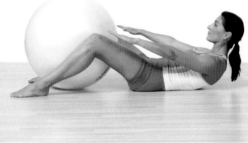

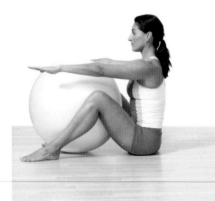

① Lie on the floor with your knees bent, ball between your legs, feet flat on the floor, arms above your head on the floor.

② Press your lower back gently into the floor and bring your arms down to your sides. Then, while squeezing your knees against the ball, slowly curl your upper body forward.

③ Come up and, as you get to the top, keep your back straight and stop when it's perpendicular to the floor.

Slowly roll down (this is hard, too!). Do this 8 times. Rest, then repeat.

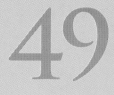

On the Floor:
Leg Pull Hamstring Curl

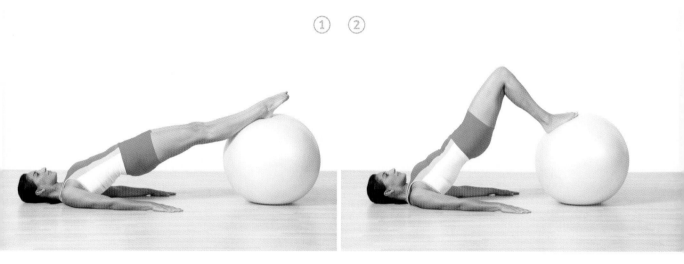

① Lie on the floor with your feet on the top of the ball, legs extended, arms by your sides, torso long and straight. Keep your shoulders away from your ears.

② Press your feet into the ball and begin to bend your knees, rolling the ball in toward your butt.

Roll it out. Do this 4 times.

This is a really tough exercise. You might only be able to do a few when you start. You'll feel it right in the center of the back of your thigh. It's really effective, so try to work up to the full set of repetitions.

On the Floor: Oblique Twist

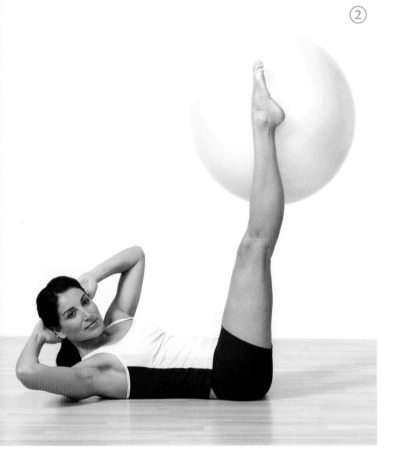

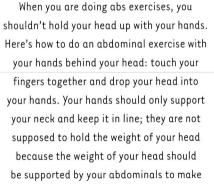

① Lie on the floor, back pressed gently onto the floor. Your legs are straight up from the hips, knees straight but not locked, hands behind your head, elbows out to the sides.

② On an exhale, lift your head, neck, and shoulders up from the floor and, as you reach the top of the move, turn your upper body toward the right. Do not clench, instead move smoothly.

Without rolling down, stay off your shoulder and repeat 8 times on each side.

When you are doing abs exercises, you shouldn't hold your head up with your hands. Here's how to do an abdominal exercise with your hands behind your head: touch your fingers together and drop your head into your hands. Your hands should only support your neck and keep it in line; they are not supposed to hold the weight of your head because the weight of your head should be supported by your abdominals to make the exercise more effective.

On the Floor: Pelvic Peel

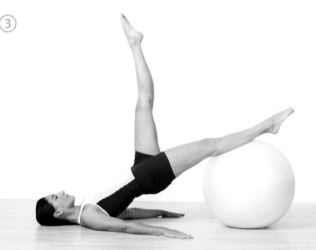

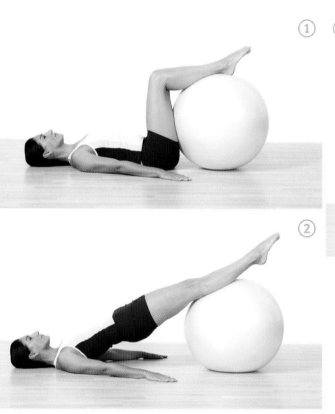

This is called a "peel" instead of a raise or lift because you should move very slowly away from the floor—creating a space between your vertebrae disks—and also lower yourself slowly back toward the floor. Part of the challenge in Pilates comes from not allowing momentum to take away from the control and precision you need to do an exercise.

(1) With the ball on the floor, lie with your hips in front of it, lower legs on the top, knees bent, back flat against the floor, abs contracted, shoulders away from the ears, arms by your sides. Your neck should be long against the floor.

(2) Slowly raise your torso, beginning from your hips and lower spine until your torso is off the floor. The ball will roll a little under your legs.

(3) At the top of the move, raise your leg to hip level and then back down. Do this slowly and with a lot of control. Rest at the bottom and then return to the start position.

Do this 4 times.

52 On the Floor: The Roll Over

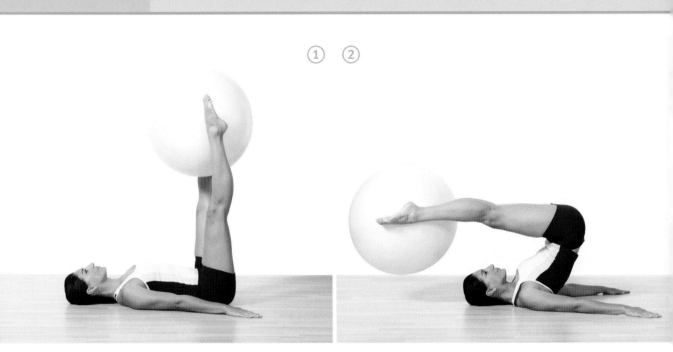

① ②

① Lie on your back, feet in the air with toes pointed, ball between your feet and lower legs. Your neck should be long against the floor, chin tilted down slightly, shoulders away from your ears. Your legs should be straight, your arms along your sides on the floor.

② Lift your hips and legs off the floor and bring your legs back over your head (this is a variation of the Plough in yoga). Then, very slowly, lower your legs back down to the start position.

Do this 4 times.

This is perhaps the hardest move in the book. If you can't do it (and believe me, you really might not be able to) focus on doing this variation: From the start position, bring your legs back toward your head, but don't lift your hips up. Instead, just bring your legs from over your head to about 45 degrees toward the floor. This will strengthen the abdominal muscles. Through the exercise, try to keep your lower back with its natural curve and braced so that all your core muscles are developing strength.

On the Floor:
Scissors Twist with Legs

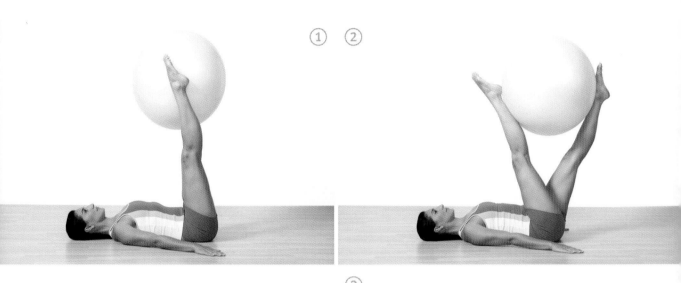

① ②

③

① Lie on the floor with your legs straight up in the air, ball between your feet and shins. Your arms should be along your sides, your neck should be long and your lower back should be pressed gently into the floor, abs contracted.

② Without moving any of your upper body, twist your legs from one side to the other. You'll feel this in your abdominals and thighs. Be sure to keep your shoulders away from your ears and your neck against the floor. Don't clench your hands or use them to hold your back down on the floor.

Do this 4 times.

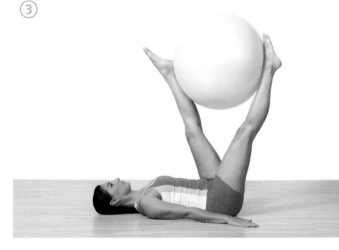

This movement requires a lot of ab strength, because you don't want to let your legs sag or your back off the floor. It's more tiring than it looks!

54

On the Floor:
Single Leg Hamstring Curl

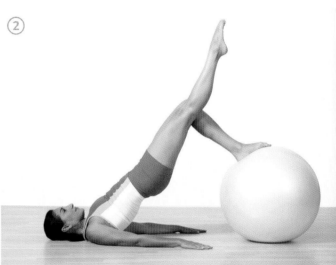

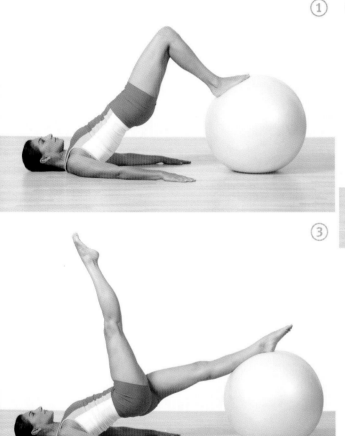

① Lie with the ball on the floor, feet on the ball, arms by your sides. Your torso and legs should be in an angle from the floor to the ball, abs contracted, butt not sagging.

② Straighten your right leg up and hold it parallel to your left leg as you roll the ball in toward your hips. This is the start position.

③ Now start the exercise: Roll the ball out with your left leg as you stretch your right leg higher, away from the ball. Be sure your abs stay contracted and your hips stay high. Pull the ball back in with your foot and roll our spine back down to the floor.

Return to the start position. Do this 4 times.

Eat protein at every meal. It builds muscle and muscle burns fat. Plus, protein is another important tool your body needs to help stabilize blood sugar levels.

On the Floor: Single Leg Stretch

①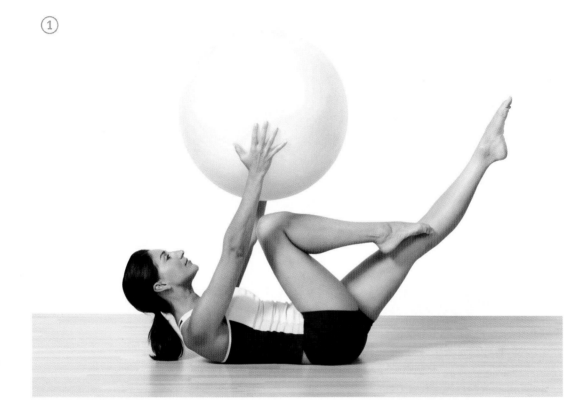

① Lie on your back with the ball in your hands, above your torso. Press your lower back gently into the floor as you raise your legs to a 45-degree angle from your hips. Keeping your shoulders away from your ears, raise your head, neck, and shoulders off the floor. Bend your right knee and bring it in toward your chest. The ball should be just above your knee. Hold this position for two counts, then switch legs continuously without moving your upper body and hips. Alternate legs up to 8 times each.

56

Leaning on Ball:
Back Leg Lift Pulses

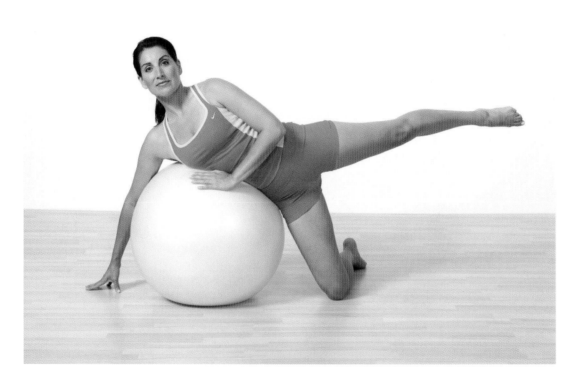

① Lie with your torso draped over the ball, right hand on the floor, left hand on the ball. Your right knee should be bent, resting on the floor.

② Keeping your hips straight, lift your left leg to hip height. This is your starting position.

③ Swing your leg back behind you and lift your leg up just a few inches.

This is an exercise that you can do without much warm-up and especially as you're watching TV. You can do an endless number of these, too, as they are working a small muscle that doesn't tire easily.

Seated on Ball: Abdominal Curl with Arm Circles

57

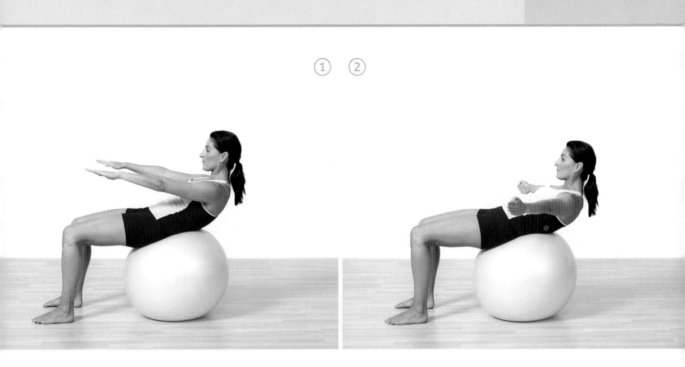

① ②

①   With the ball on the floor, lie on the top, feet on the floor, knees bent. Your arms should be out from your body, long and straight, parallel to the floor. Your shoulders should be away from your ears, back with a natural curve.

②   On an exhale, roll down slightly as you contract your abs. Your back should be fully supported by the ball, up to your shoulders. As you do this, bring your arms back around your head in a big circle. This will cause the abs to work harder for another second or two.

Come down to start. Do this 8 times.

58 Seated on Ball: Abdominal Curl with Arm Reach

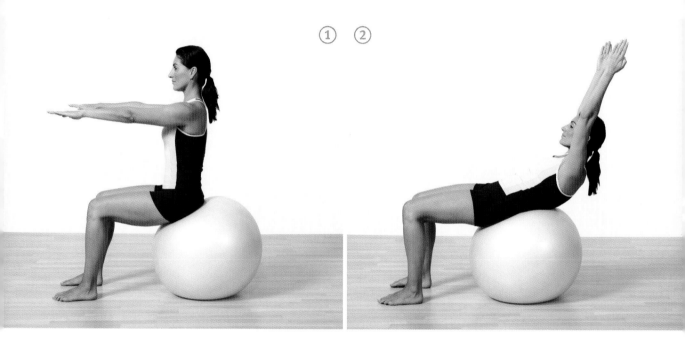

① ②

① With the ball on the floor, sit on the top, feet on the floor, knees bent. Your arms should be out from your body, long and straight, parallel to the floor. Your shoulders should be away from your ears, back with a natural curve.

② On an exhale, roll down as you contract your abs. Your back should be fully supported by the ball, up to your shoulders. Your arms should move alongside your ears, high. Now, roll up to the start position on top of the ball.

Come down to start. Do this 4 times.

Seated on Ball: Abdominal Curl with Single Arm Reach Back

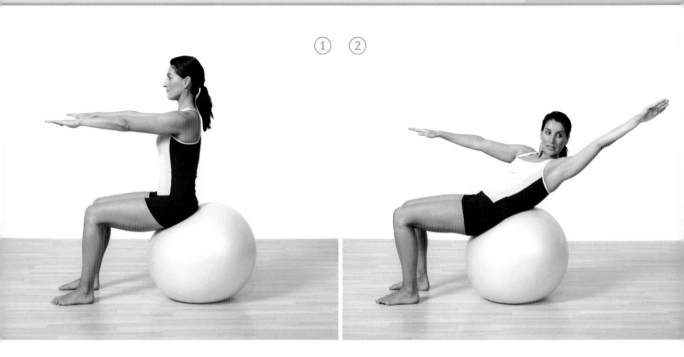

(1) With the ball on the floor, sit on the top, feet on the floor, knees bent. Your arms should be out from your body, long and straight, parallel to the floor. Your shoulders should be away from your ears, back with a natural curve.

(2) On an exhale, roll down as you contract your abs. Your back should be fully supported by the ball, up to your shoulders. As you do this, keep your right arm straight in front of your body. Bring your left arm back behind your body in a torso twist. This will cause a release in your core as you hold the contraction longer.

Roll up to a seated position on the ball. Do this 8 times on each side.

60 Seated on Ball: Abdominal Curl Up

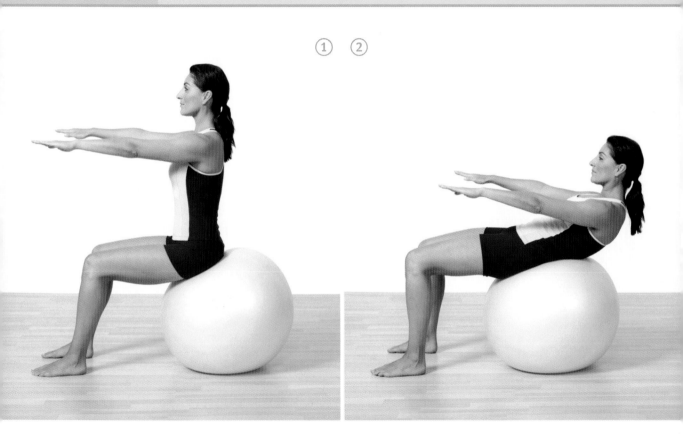

① ②

(1) With the ball on floor, sit on the top.

(2) Slide down about 6 inches, so that your butt is just below the apex of the ball. Your feet should be flat on the floor, knees bent, feet under knees, arms extended in front of your body. Your head, neck, and shoulders are off the ball in a contraction of your abs.

(3) Keeping your feet still, roll the ball behind you as you raise your head, neck, and shoulders up to a seated position. Be sure to keep your elbows down and your abs contracted.

Come back down slowly. Do this 8 times.

Seated on Ball: Core Twist

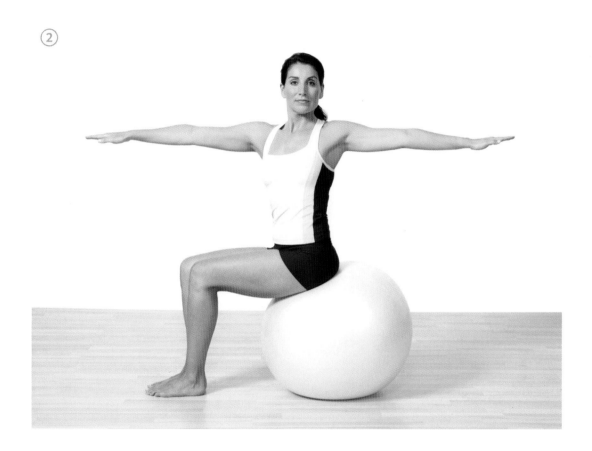

① With the ball on the floor, sit on the top, feet on the floor, knees bent. Your arms should be out from your body, long and straight, parallel to the floor. Your shoulders should be away from your ears, back with a natural curve.

② On an exhale, turn to your right side without raising your shoulders or moving your hips. Inhale. Come back to center, then exhale and turn to the left.

Do this 8 times on each side.

62

Seated on Ball: Front Arm Raises with Dumbbells

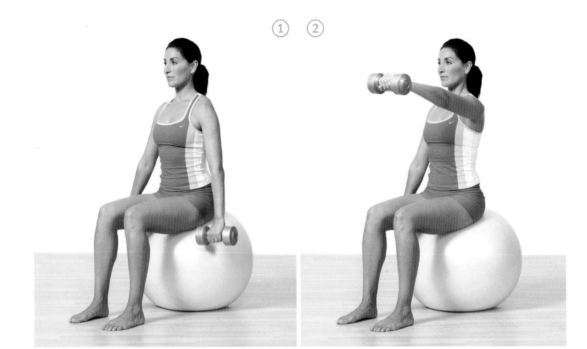

① ②

① With the ball on the floor, sit on the top, holding a dumbbell in each hand. Keep your shoulders relaxed, chin slightly pointed down, crown of the head up facing the ceiling. Your arms are long and hands are resting in front of the ball.

② Raise your right arm to shoulder height without raising your shoulder toward your ear and keeping your abs contracted. Lower the weight down and repeat with the left arm.

Do this 8 times with each arm.

The deltoid has three aspects or sides: the anterior (front shoulder), posterior (back shoulder), and medial (middle). It's best to work the shoulder in all its directions (remember, it's a ball and socket joint, like the hips, which means you can move your arm in a full circle) to keep it strong and healthy. That's why we do raises and presses in all directions.

Seated on Ball: Lateral Arm Raises with Dumbbells

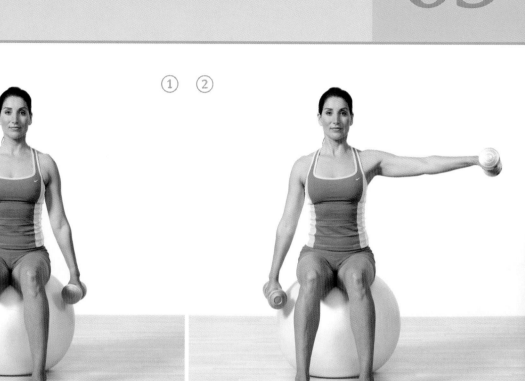

(1) With the ball on the floor, sit on the top with a dumbbell in each hand. Keep your shoulders relaxed, your chin pointed slightly down, crown of the head facing the ceiling.

(2) Without moving any other part of your body, raise your right arm out to the side, keeping the shoulder down.

Lower the weight down and repeat on the other side. Do this 8 times with each arm.

64 Seated on Ball: Overhead Shoulder Press with Dumbbells

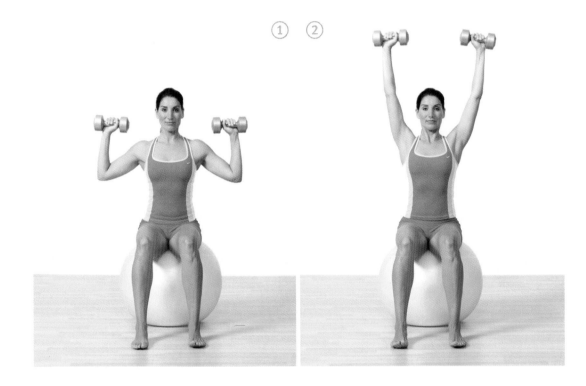

① ②

① With the ball on the floor, sit on the top, feet on the floor, knees bent, arms out from your sides, a dumbbell in each hand, elbows bent at right angles, hands just outside of your ears.

② Keeping your shoulders down, straighten your elbows and raise your hands up without locking your elbows.

Come back to the start position. Do this 8 times.

Why do I keep mentioning that you should keep your shoulders down? Because many people hunch their shoulders up, especially when they exercise, and that takes away from the effectiveness of the program. If your shoulders are in the proper position, then the muscles can do their job. So always be conscious of relaxing your shoulders; this will not only take away any feelings of tension you have, but it will give you better posture and make you fitter, too.

Seated on Ball: Rotator Cuff

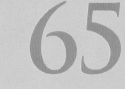

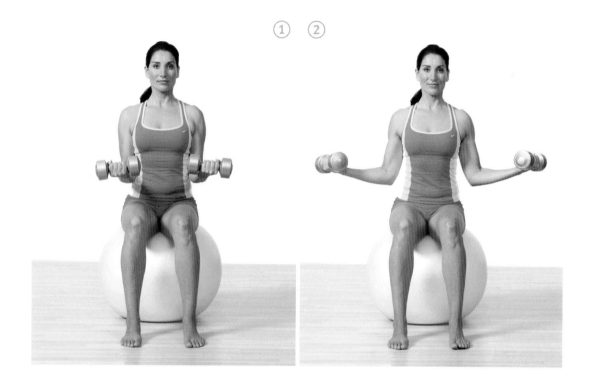

① Sit on the ball holding a dumbbell in each hand, shoulders relaxed, neck long. Keep your elbows bent and close to your sides, almost squeezing the tops of your arms into your sides. Your forearms should be parallel to the floor, elbows bent.

② Moving only your forearms, bring them out to your sides. Make sure your shoulders and upper arms stay still.

Do this 8 times.

66 Seated on Ball: The Sevens

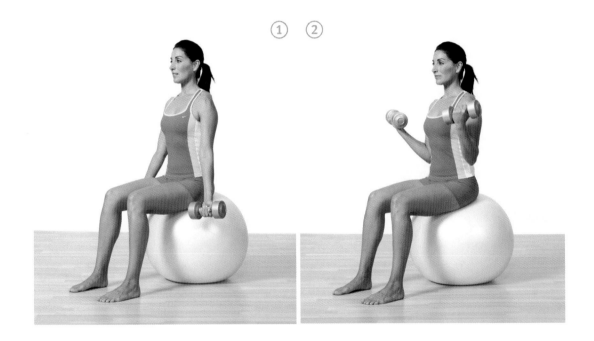

This exercise has three parts—you're going to do each part of the move 7 times.

① First, sit on the ball with a dumbbell in each hand. With your arms down, keep your elbows close to your sides and your shoulders relaxed away from your ears. Start with your elbows bent, forearms parallel to the floor.

② Now, bring your hands up toward your shoulders without moving your upper arms. Lower to the start position. Do this 7 times.

③ Next, start with your forearms parallel again, but lower your arm to an almost straight position. Do this 7 times with each arm.

④ Finally, do the full range of motion, moving from a mostly straight arm to bringing your hand close to your shoulder. Do this 7 times.

This exercise works the biceps muscles, which run on the front of the arm.

Seated on Ball: Single Leg Extension and Twist

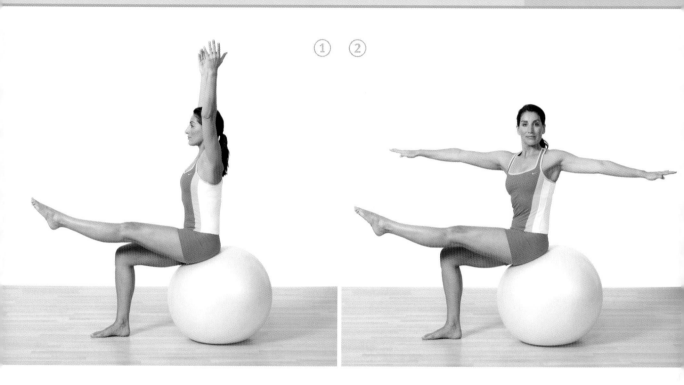

① ②

① Sit on the ball with a natural curve in your lower back, knees bent, feet on the floor. Keep your arms above your head, shoulders relaxed, and your torso tall. Straighten the knee of your left leg and bring your lower leg up so that your entire leg is pointed slightly up. Don't lock your knee.

② As you straighten your left leg, turn to your left, bringing your arms down to shoulder height, and twist in your torso. Your upper body should remain straight and long. The movement should feel like a rotation or corkscrew, your hips should be still.

Come back to center and go to the left. Do this 8 times on each side.

68

Seated on Ball: Triceps Overhead Extension with Dumbbells

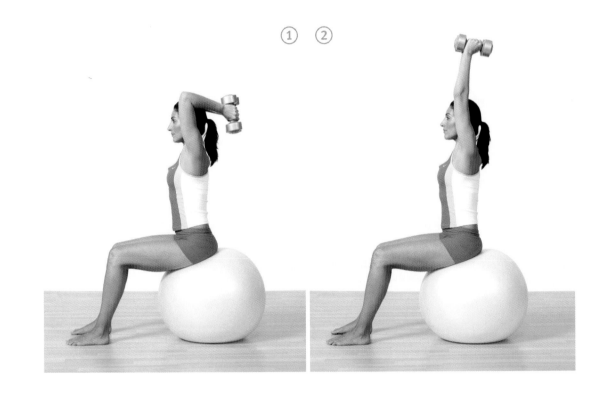

① ②

① Sit on the ball with a dumbbell in each hand, shoulders relaxed. Raise your arms over your head and put the dumbbells behind your head, elbows bent by your ears. Do not hunch up with your shoulders.

② Now, raise your hands and the dumbbells to an almost straight-arm position, stopping short of locking your elbows. You should feel your triceps muscle contract. If not, use a heavier weight (you can go up to eight pounds most likely). Lower your arms.

Seated on Ball: Side Sevens

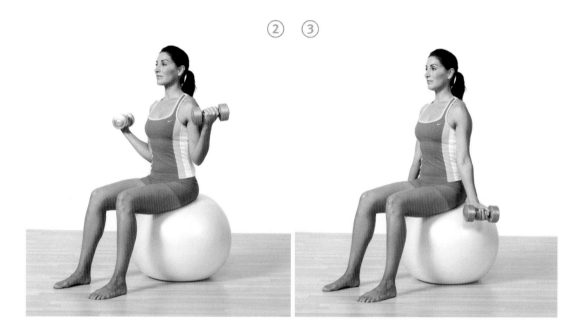

This exercise has three parts—you're going to do each part of the move 7 times.

① First, sit on the ball with a dumbbell in each hand. With your arms down, keep your elbows close to your sides and your shoulders relaxed away from your ears. Start with your elbows bent, forearms parallel to the floor. This time, your arms are turned out to the sides from your shoulders.

② Now, bring your hands up toward your shoulders without moving your upper arms. Lower to the start position. Do this 7 times.

③ Next, start with your forearms parallel again, but lower your arm to an almost straight position. Do this 7 times.

④ Finally, do the full range of motion, moving from a mostly straight arm to bringing your hand close to your shoulder. Do this 7 times.

As you can tell by their name, the biceps are two muscles. Doing "Sevens" plus "Side Sevens" work both parts.

70

Leaning on Ball:
Front Leg Lift Pulses

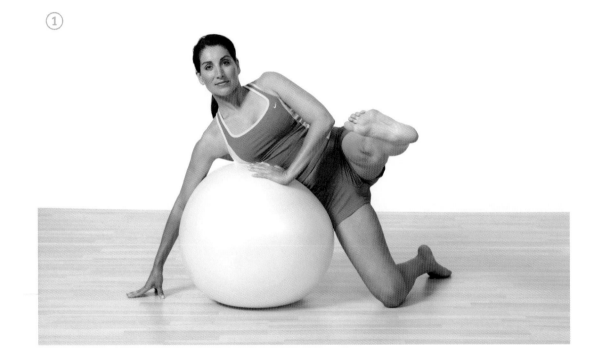

① Lie with your torso draped over the ball, right hand on the floor, left hand on the ball. Your right knee should be bent, resting on the floor.

② Keeping your hips straight, lift your left leg to hip height and bring it in front of your body. This is your starting position.

③ Now, lift your leg up a few inches (it won't be able to go very high) with your foot flexed. Come back to start.

We are working the same muscles with different exercises, which means that, as we go on, each move will feel harder and the reps will get more difficult to finish. You can always take a break, stretch your leg out, and start again. As you get these exercises down, you can rearrange their order in the way that works best for you. Remember, pain is not an indication of effectiveness, but you should feel a sense of tiredness in your muscles toward the end of your repetitions.

Standing Back Lunge

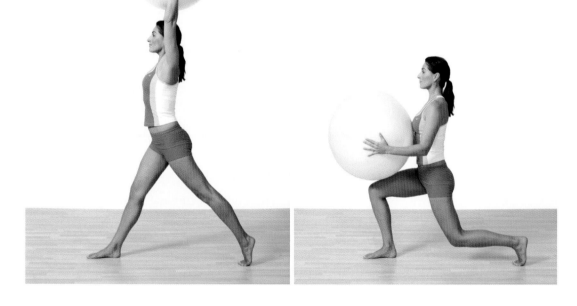

(1) Come to the start position with feet together, ball in front of your torso. Step back about three feet with your right foot. The back foot starts with the leg straight. Stay on the ball of your foot the whole time.

(2) Bend both knees, being sure to keep your front knee from going past your toes and lowering your back knee until just above the floor. Do not lean your torso forward or back. Keep it centered over your legs.

Return to the start position. Do this 8 times with each leg.

To make this and other lunges really tough, keep the ball above your head throughout the exercise.

72 Standing Front Lunge

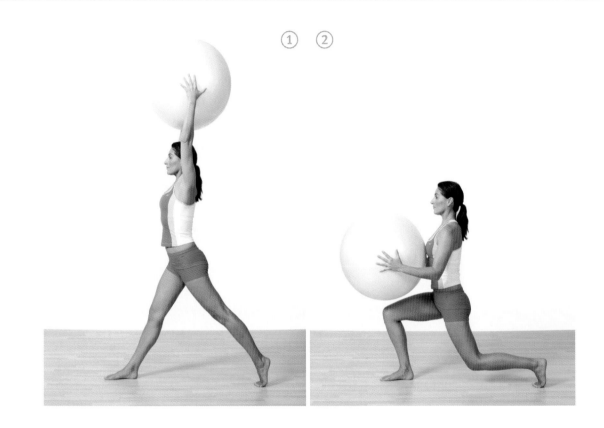

① ②

① Stand with your right foot about three to four feet ahead of your left, torso centered over both legs. Hold the ball over your head, as high as possible while keeping your shoulders relaxed.

② Without leaning forward, bend your knees. Your rear knee should be just above the floor while your front knee should not go past your toes. As you come down, bring the ball to your chest.

Do this 8 times with each leg.

The lunge is another perfect exercise, meaning it works a large number of muscles in very effective ways. The front leg gets its quadriceps and glute muscles strengthened, while the back leg gets a stretch in the hip flexor and quadriceps.

Standing Squats Holding Ball

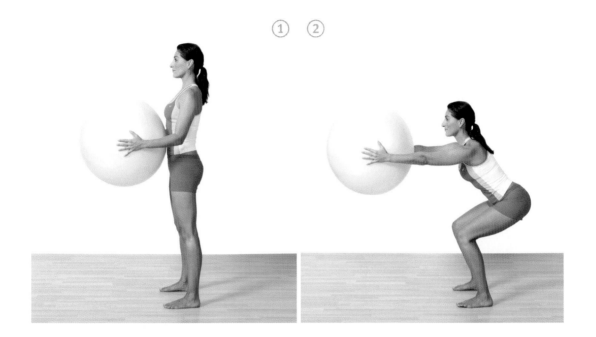

① ②

① Stand with your feet hip-width apart, holding the ball in front of your torso. Keeping your back straight, bend from your hips as if you're sitting on a chair. As you move into the squat, move the ball away from your body so that your arms end being perpendicular to the floor.

② As you come up, squeeze your butt at the top of the move.

Do this quickly, one count as you come up, one count as you go down. Repeat 8 times.

The squat strengthens and sculpts the butt, hamstrings, quadriceps, and calves and it has a million variations. Once you have this traditional move down, you can do it with your feet wide apart and turned out (as in a second-position plié), with your heels together and feet turned out in a first-position plié (you won't come down very far because this challenges your balance a lot), or you can keep your legs wide apart but in parallel position and try to raise one leg as you come up (this is a sumo squat).

74 Standing Wall Calf Raises

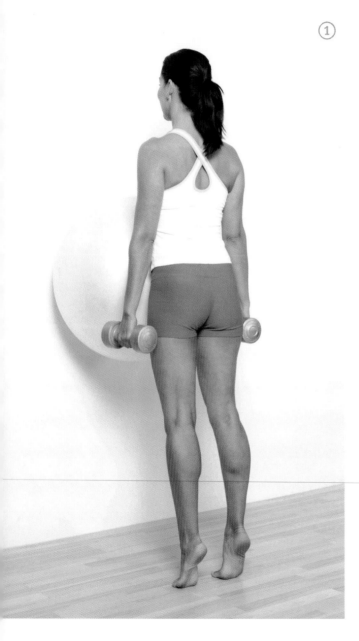

(1) (1) With the ball against the wall, stand with your belly against the ball, a dumbbell in each hand. Keeping your shoulders down, raise up onto your toes.

Hold this position for two counts, then lower down. Do this 8 times.

Standing Wall Leg Lift Sides

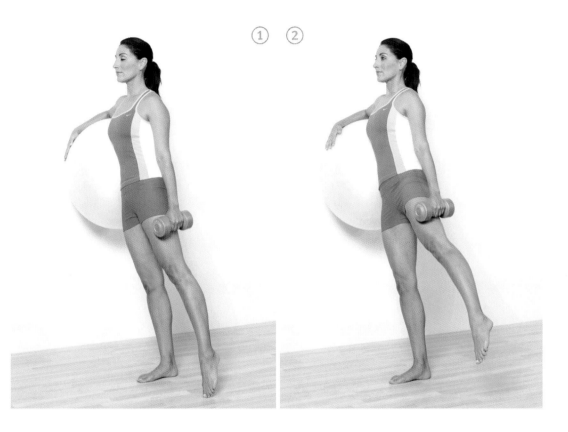

① ②

① Stand with the ball against the wall, right side of your body against the ball, right arm over the ball, hand near the wall. Hold a dumbbell in your left hand against the outside of your thigh. Your right leg is next to the ball and your left leg is facing forward, toes pointed. All your weight is on your right leg. Be sure your abs are contracted and your shoulders are relaxed.

② With your torso in a natural curve, lift your outside leg and raise it to a height that is a long extension but that doesn't force you to change the level of your hip. Then lower your leg.

Do this slowly without letting momentum take over. Do this 8 times on each side.

76

Standing Wall Lunge Front: Triceps Kick-Back

① ②

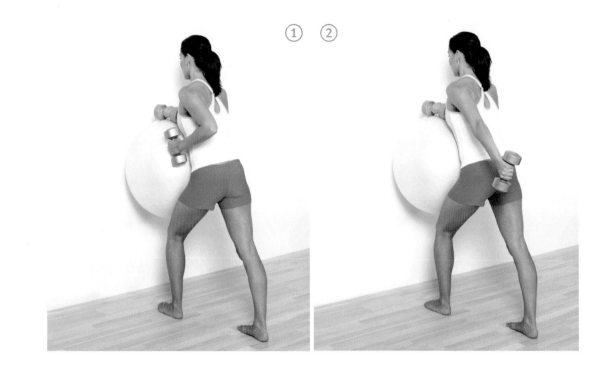

① With the ball against the wall, reaching from your ribs to your thighs, stand against it, holding a dumbbell in each hand. Put your left leg under the ball and your right leg back, as if in a partial lunge. Put your right hand on the top of the ball and hold your left arm with a bent elbow, weight just near the ball.

② Keeping your shoulders down, extend your left arm, trying not to lock your elbow when it's straight.

Do this 8 times with each arm.

◎

If you notice your muscles are getting strong and toned but you still feel unhappy with your weight, try changing your diet for a few weeks to lose a couple of pounds. You might find that your eating habits are keeping your new, long, sleek muscles covered with a little too much fat to see a difference in your shape.

Standing Wall Lunge Front: Reverse Fly with Dumbbells

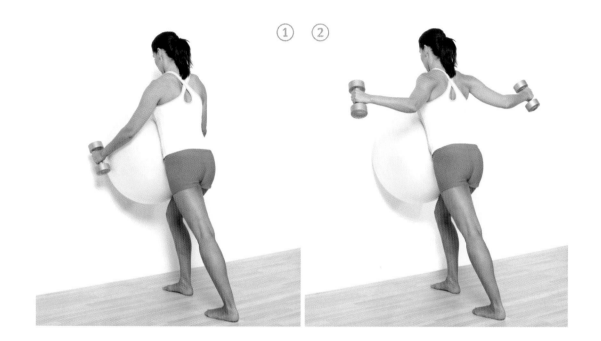

① With the ball at chest level, press it against the wall, holding a dumbbell in each hand. Step back with your left leg at an angle, while keeping your right foot on the floor directly under the ball. Your arms should be straight across the ball on both sides with the dumbbells close to the wall. You can squeeze the ball a bit with your body so it doesn't roll.

② Now start the exercise: Squeeze your shoulder blades together. Then, keeping your shoulders down, bend your elbows and bring your arms back until your hands are at your hips and your elbows are way past your back. Return to the start position.

Do this 8 times.

It's always a good idea to stretch a muscle after you've done an exercise to strengthen it. Studies have shown that stretching after resistance exercise actually builds strength faster than not stretching—and stronger muscles burn more calories than weaker ones!

78

Standing Wall Lunge Front: Single Arm Row with Dumbbells

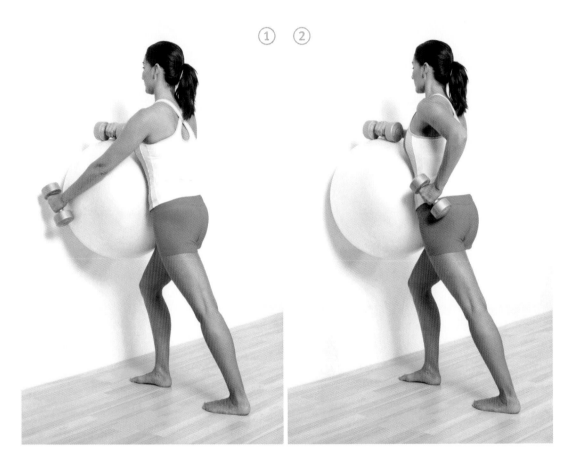

① Stand with the ball against the wall at torso height. Put your right leg under the ball with a bent knee. Your left leg should be back, straight from your hip. Your right arm should be resting on the ball, holding a dumbbell. Your left arm should be down pointing toward the wall.

② Keeping your neck long and your shoulders down, bend your elbow and bring your hand in toward your hip. Return to the start position.

Do this 8 times with each arm.

Standing Wall Overhead Shoulder Press with Calf Raises Dumbbells

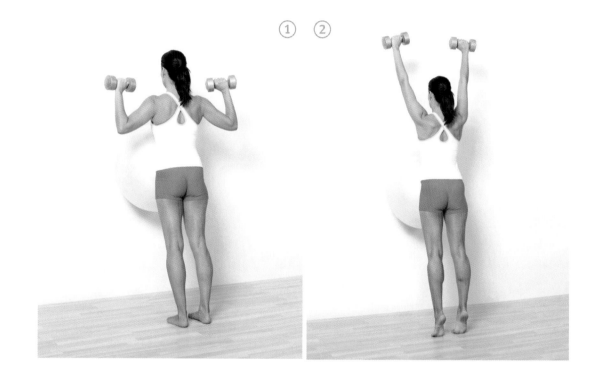

① With the ball against the wall, stand with your belly pressed against it, legs out on a slight angle, feet on the floor, a few inches apart. Hold a weight in each hand, elbows bent, hands by your ears. Be sure to keep your shoulders relaxed and your abs contracted.

② Straighten your elbows and raise your arms over your head without scrunching your shoulders up. As you do this, come up on your toes. Come back down to start.

Do this 8 times.

⊚

The shoulders aren't large muscles and most women can only lift, at most, about 10 pounds. But don't worry, even light weights will make a big difference in how strong, healthy, and sexy your shoulders become.

80

Standing Wall Overhead Shoulder Press with Squat Holding Dumbbells

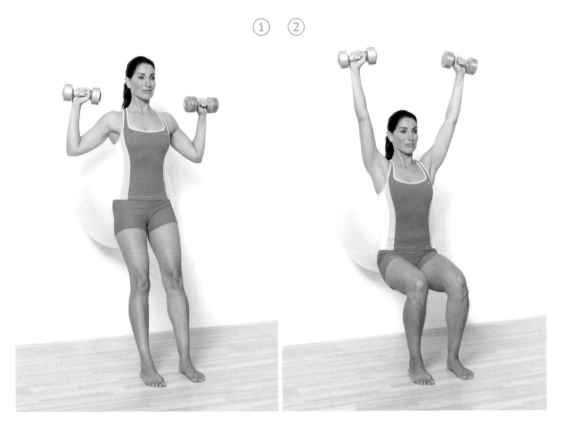

① ②

① With the ball against the wall, press your back gently against it, a dumbbell in each hand, arms raised, elbows bent, legs angled out from your hips. Keep your abs contracted.

② Keeping your back straight and your neck long and without raising your shoulders, bend your knees as you straighten your arms. Come down until your thighs are parallel to the floor and your arms are straight, but not locked. The ball will roll with you.

Come back to the start position. Do this 8 times.

Standing Wall Overhead Triceps Extensions with Dumbbells

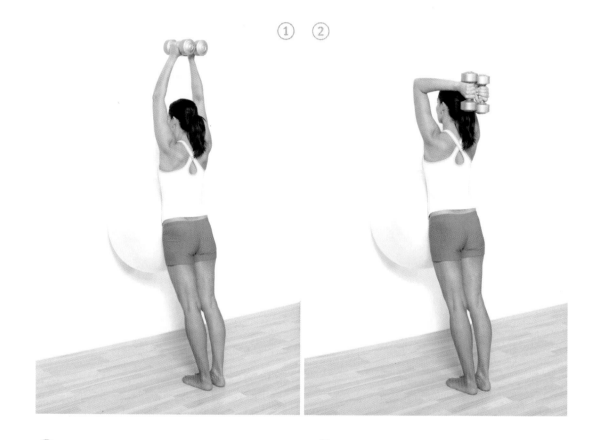

① ②

① With the ball against the wall between from your ribs and your thighs, stand against it, holding your arms up straight over your head, a dumbbell in each hand. Keep your legs and feet together.

② Slowly bend your elbows and let your hands drop behind your head. Do this without raising your shoulders or letting your hands fall too fast. Straighten your elbows and raise your hands back up.

Do this 8 times.

82

Standing Wall Prances

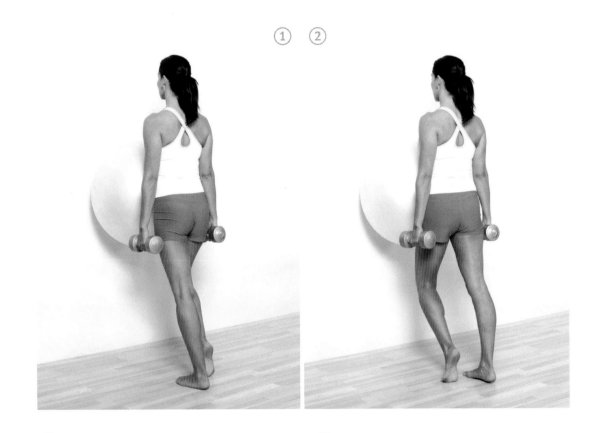

① ②

① With the ball against the wall, stand in front of it with your belly and chest against it, a dumbbell in each hand, shoulders down, abs contracted, back long. Your legs should be out in a slight angle from the ball, starting from your hips, heels on the floor.

② Without moving your upper body, pick up the heel of one foot, then quickly lower it down as you pick up the heel of the other foot. Prances go very quickly, but the rest of your body should stay still.

Do this 32 times (16 times with each foot).

Standing Wall Push-Ups

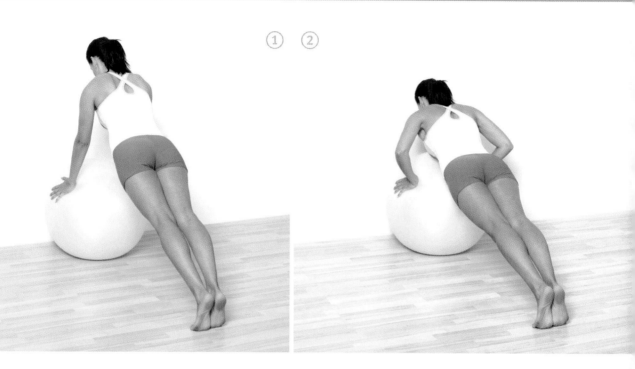

(1)   (2)

(1) Put the ball against the wall and on the floor, with your hands on the top and toward the side. Keep your body at an angle and your feet on the floor, legs straight. Your arms should be straight but not locked.

(2) Bend your elbows and come down into a push-up, elbows going out to the sides. Be sure your abs are contracted and your butt is in line with your back and not sticking up in the air. The wider you place your hands on the ball, the easier it will feel. Come back to the start position.

Do this 8 times.

This is a traditional push-up made much harder because you are using the ball, which means you have to balance and use your core muscles. To make this easier, you can come down to your knees. To make it harder? Take the ball away from the wall and try to keep it steady as you do your push-ups. **That** is really hard!

84 Standing Wall Single Leg Squat with Dumbbells

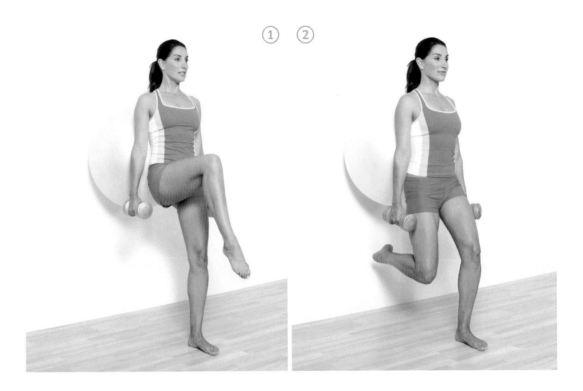

① ②

① With the ball against the wall, stand against it, holding a dumbbell in each hand. Your chin should be parallel to the floor, neck long, abs contracted. Bring your right knee up and get balanced on your left leg.

② Now, to start the exercise, bring your right leg back, knee bent, and begin to bend your left knee into a squat. The ball will roll with you. Come back to the start position.

Do this 4 times with each leg.

◎

Go to sleep. Get enough rest. Your body needs time to recover from daily stress and your workouts. If you are exhausted your body simply can't perform well. And much worse, you're more prone to injury if you don't get enough rest.

Standing Wall Leg Lift Rear

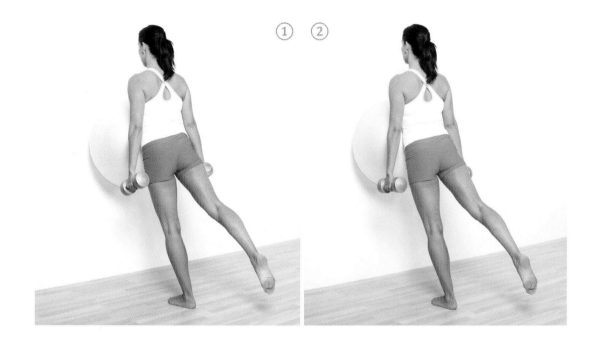

① 　②

① Stand with the ball against the wall and lean against it with your chest and abs. Hold a dumbbell in each hand. Be sure your shoulders are relaxed.

② Raise your right leg behind you, but not so much that your hips go out of alignment (they should stay level and even throughout this exercise).

③ Now, raise your right leg higher, once again, not so high that your hips aren't even. You won't be able to bring your leg very high but you should feel your glute muscle tense. Lower your leg.

There are three gluteal muscles: the gluteus maximus, gluteus medius, and the gluteus minimus. Squats and lunges work the maximus, but the medius and minimus are worked by smaller exercises. By "smaller" I mean that you use a smaller range of motion. And any move in which you lift your leg, such as this one, also works the medius and minimus. These muscles are underused and weak in most people, which is why you feel the move's effectiveness so quickly. The rewards of these moves are great, because you'll see a real "lift" in your butt from doing them.

86 Standing Wall Pliés with Dumbbells

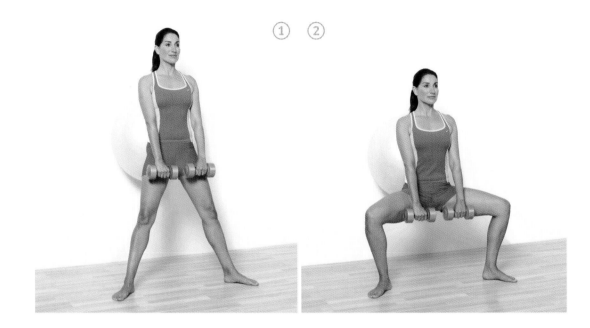

① ②

① Put the ball against the wall at the middle of your lower back and lean against it. Hold a dumbbell in each hand. Stand with your torso straight, abs contracted, and put your feet into second position—your feet should be wide apart, toes turned out. Watch your knees—they stay on track over toes. Be sure to turn out from your hips, not your knees.

② Keeping your torso straight, bend your knees into a deep plié. Contrary to what you would imagine, the ball will roll up your back against the wall.

Come back to the start position. Do this 4 times.

Pilates—and some of my exercises—use dance positions for arm and leg placement. Ballet requires dancers to hold their bodies in awkward positions that look beautiful (but are difficult). *Port de bras* means carriage of the arms in French and it describes the movement of the arms in ballet. To hold your arms properly (and really strengthen your upper back and the backs of your arms) make a circle with your arms in front of your body at shoulder height. Now, slightly lift the backs of your arms (the triceps) while dropping your shoulders. You should feel the movement in your upper back, too.

Walking Lunges

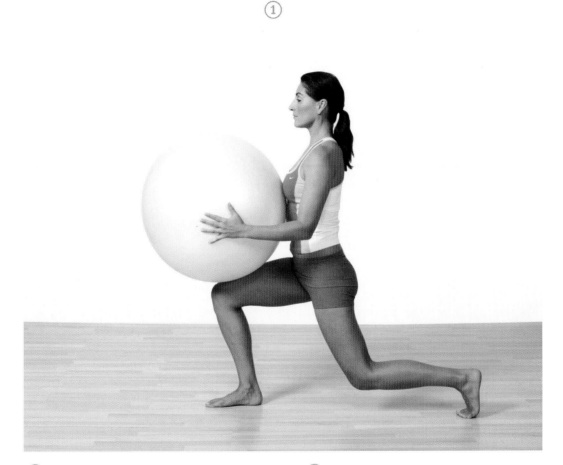

(1) Standing with your feet together, hold the ball with both hands in front of your torso. Take a wide step forward with your right foot, and bend your knees as your foot lands. Make sure your leading knee doesn't go past your toe.

(2) Come up to a standing position as you bring your left foot forward past your right to go into the next step of the lunge.

Do this 16 times (8 times with each leg.)

88

Wall Squat

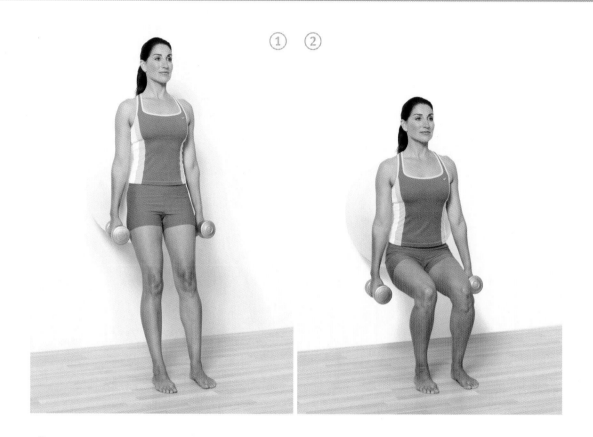

① Put the ball against a wall and put your back against the ball (it should reach from just below your shoulders to just above your hips). Hold a dumbbell in each hand. Your legs should be on a slight angle from the ball.

② Start to go into a squat. The ball will roll down the wall with you and you should come to a position in which your thighs are pointed slightly down.

Come back to the start position. Do this 8 times.

The Stretches

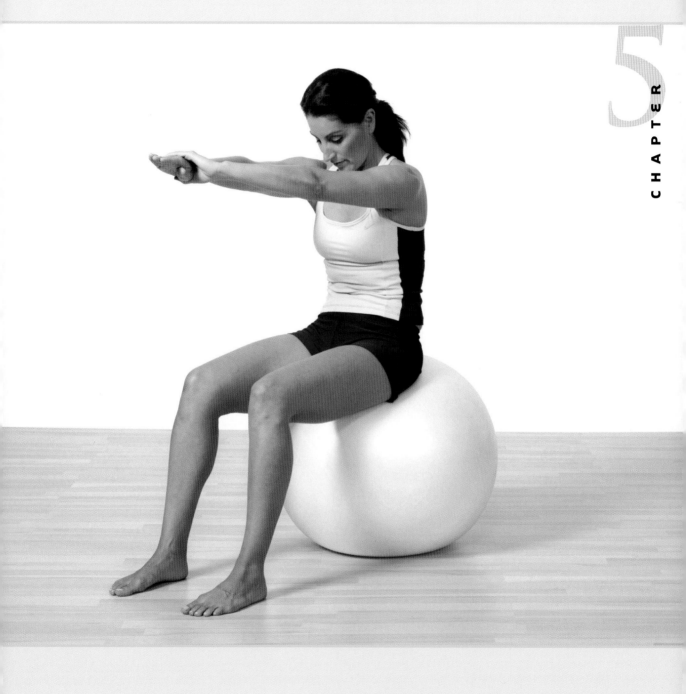

CHAPTER 5

89

Lay Back Over Ball: Open Chest Stretch

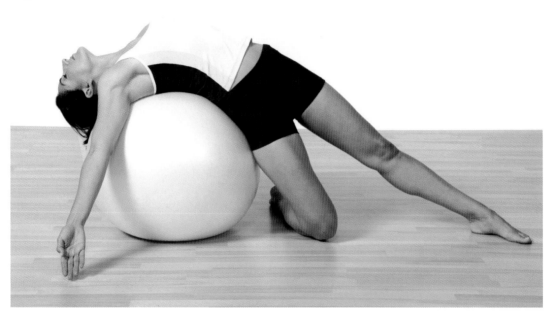

① With the ball on the floor, lie over the top with your chest and shoulders supported, head relaxed down the top slope of the ball. Bend your right leg and rest your weight on your right knee and shin, while extending your left leg long, foot on the floor.

② On an exhale, roll toward your right, letting your arms extend down the side of the ball and feeling your chest open and stretch against the top of the ball.

Keep your shoulders down from your ears and your hips long in the front of your body.

◎

You can stretch any part of your body by letting it hang over the top of the ball. Some variations on this stretch include putting your lower torso on top (you might have to hold yourself up by putting your hands on the floor), laying your side over the top (this will stretch the side of your body facing the ceiling), and lying on your front torso to stretch your back.

On the Floor:
Straddle Stretch to the Side

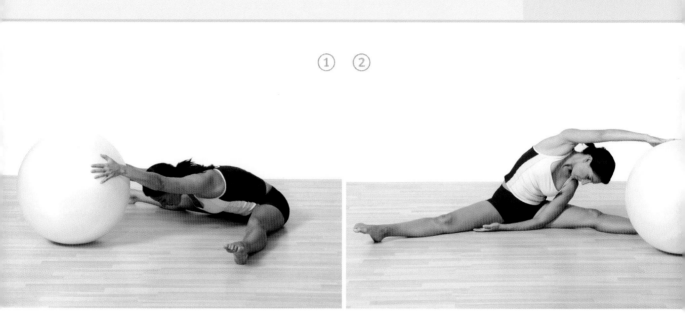

① ②

① With the ball on the floor, sit behind it, legs out in a wide V position. Put your hands on top of the ball. Be sure your butt is in contact with the floor and your thighs are rolling out a bit from your hips (your kneecaps should face the ceiling). Your back is relaxed and your shoulders are down.

② Now, roll the ball to the left with your right hand on top. As you do this, bring your left arm up and over your head, stretching the left side of your body. Be sure your butt doesn't come off the ground. If it does, relax the stretch a little. Turn your head up to increase the stretch.

91 Seated Side Lunges

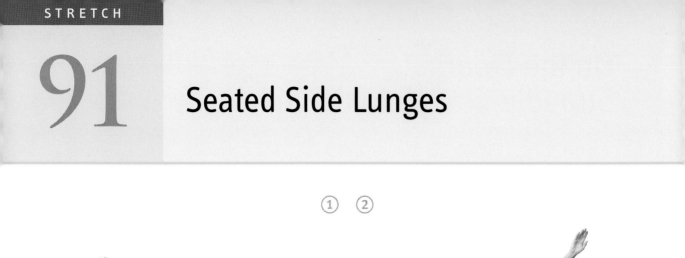

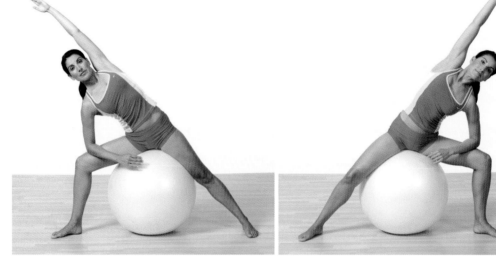

(1) Sit with the ball between your legs, which should be turned out. Bend your right knee so that you are in a side lunge. As you move your legs, tilt your torso to the right, bringing your right arm to your right knee. Raise your left arm along the left side of your torso, over your head, keeping it straight.

(2) Take two counts to come down into this posture, hold the pose for two counts, then go to the other side.

Do this 8 times on each side.

Build muscle. Incorporate resistance training exercises into your routine. By increasing your muscle to fat ratio, you will burn many more calories all day, every day. Did you know that muscle is the only tissue in the human body capable of burning fat? Adding in a few exercises only three times a week will help you reach your fitness goals.

Leaning on Ball: Shoulder Stretch

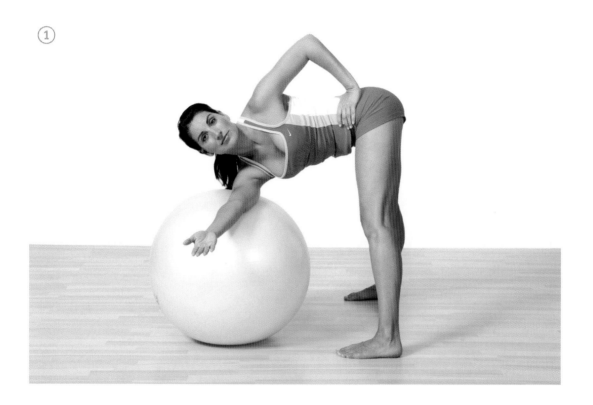

1. Stand with the ball a foot or so in front of you, feet far apart. Bend forward from your hips, right shoulder on the ball, torso twisted, left hand on your hip, back flat.

2. Roll the ball out under your shoulder as your turn toward your left. Bring your left hand to your left hip as you open your chest to the left side. Keep your legs straight, but your knees relaxed. You should feel this in your upper back, shoulder, and chest.

You'll know you're exercising hard enough if you feel slightly breathless (not so much that you have to stop to catch your breath) and if you would find it difficult to carry on a conversation while you work out. If you can easily sing along to the music you're listening to, then pick up your intensity a little.

93

Leaning on Ball:
Side Leg Kick Front and Back

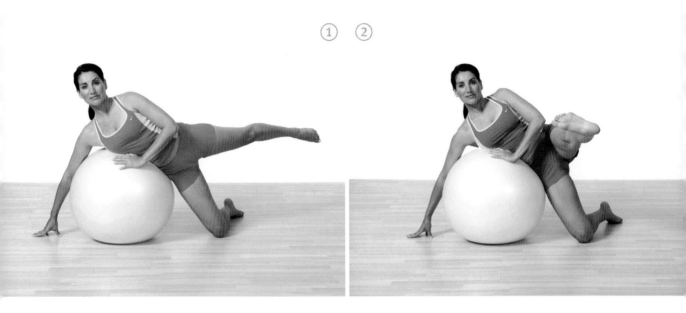

① ②

① Lie with your torso draped over the ball, right hand on the floor, left hand on the ball. Your right knee should be bent, resting on the floor.

② Keeping your hips straight, lift your left leg to hip height. This is your starting position.

③ Bring your left leg forward with foot flexed and without throwing your hips out of position. You should feel a hamstring stretch. Now, slowly swing your leg back, with a pointed foot, also without moving your butt. You should feel your butt muscle contract and your hip flexor stretch.

This exercise works on toning the butt and stretching the hamstring muscles and the hip flexor. It's a great move to do at the end of a workout because it loosens the muscles near the hip, lengthening the muscles that have worked so hard during these exercises.

On the Floor: Child's Pose

①

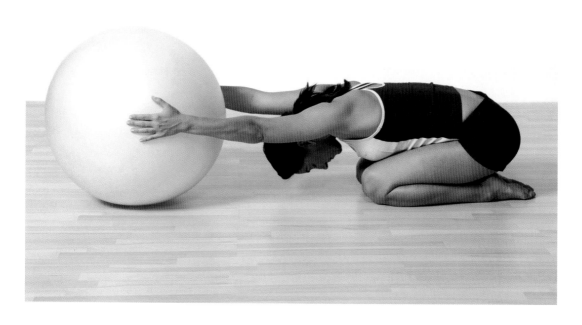

① With the ball on the floor, put your hands on top of the ball and kneel down, shins on the floor. Let your back fall through your arms as you let the ball roll away from you a bit. Feel the stretch in your low back as you pull your hips back and let your arms go in front of you.

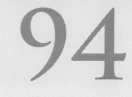

Exercise has been shown to be one of the best remedies for an aching back. If you have lower back pain or strain in your back, try taking a walk or swimming to relieve the muscle tension. Yoga has also been helpful for back problems..

95

On the Floor: Leg Straddle Wide Side Arm Reach

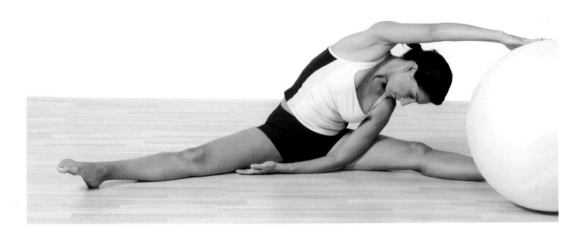

(1) With the ball on the floor, sit behind it, legs out in a wide V position. Put your hands on top of the ball. Be sure your butt is in contact with the floor and your thighs are rolling out a bit from your hips (your knee caps should face the ceiling). Your back is relaxed and your shoulders are down.

(2) Now, roll the ball to the left with your right hand on top. As you do this, bring your left arm up and over your head, stretching the left side of your body. Be sure your butt doesn't come off the ground. If it does, relax the stretch a little.

Stretching is relaxed and easy; you aren't trying to push yourself into an extreme position. Instead, you should feel a very slight pull that eases the muscles you have just worked. Work with the breath—stretch a little further on the exhale.

Seated on Ball: Chest Stretch

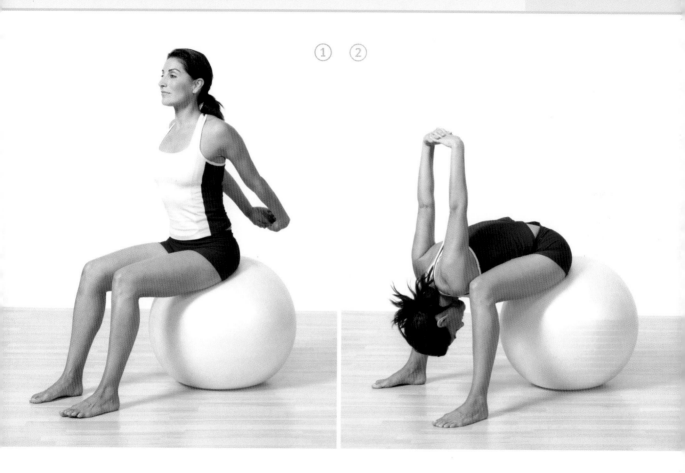

① ②

① With the ball on the floor, sit slightly below the top, feet on the floor.

② Keeping your shoulders down, clasp your hands behind your back. Breathe deeply and raise your arms above your head as you bend forward from your waist. Keep your hips on the ball even though it will roll back a bit.

Snack time? Eat whole foods, not simple sugars or salty foods. Carbohydrates aren't the main culprits in weight gain. It's the carbs from simple sugars such as candy bars and fruit juices that really lead to trouble. The higher your blood sugar the more slowly you burn fat.

97

Seated on Ball: Neck Stretch

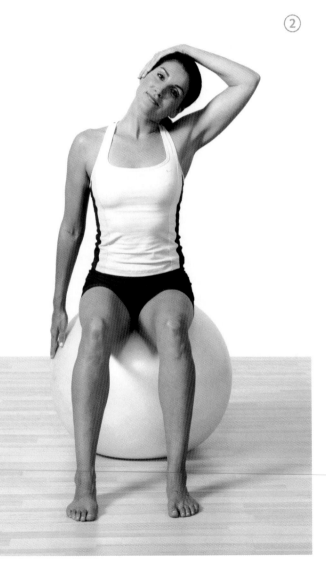

② ①

1. With the ball on the floor, sit on the top, feet on the floor, shoulders away from your ears, abs contracted. Your arms should be down by your sides.

2. Raise your left hand and put it over your head, resting your palm just above your right ear. Very gently, press your right ear into your palm, keeping your right shoulder down and relaxed. The ball and your hips shouldn't move.

After your workout, drink some water and, if you feel hungry, try eating a hard-boiled egg and maybe a banana. You don't want to eat too much, but protein will help build muscle and the banana will give you some carbs for energy, as well as some potassium, which you lose when you sweat.

Seated on Ball: Rhomboid Stretch

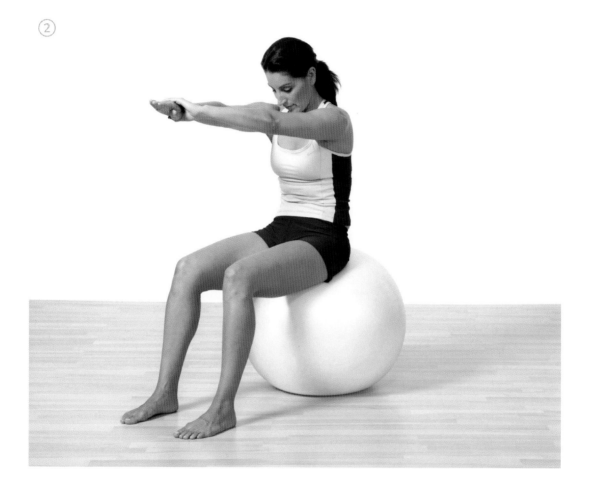

② With the ball on the floor, sit on the top, feet on the floor, abs contracted, arms by your sides, shoulders away from ears.

② Keeping your shoulder relaxed, clasp your hands in front of your body, arms long. Pull your hands forward to feel the stretch in the middle of your back. Drop your head down between your shoulders, but don't hunch up.

99

Seated on Ball: Side Stretch

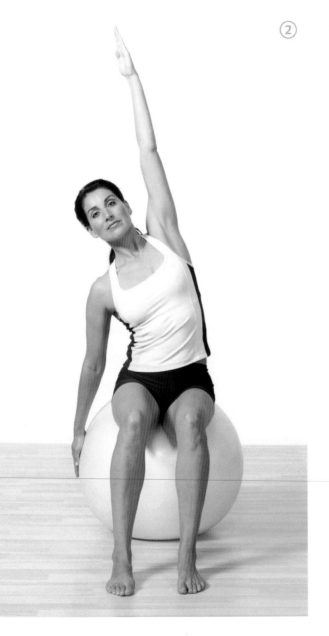

(2)

(1) With the ball on the floor, sit on the top, feet on the floor, arms by your sides, neck long, abs contracted.

(2) On an inhale, raise your left arm straight above your head, being sure to keep your shoulders down. Then, on an exhale, lean slightly to the right, creating a curve in your right side. The ball will roll a little.

(3) Come back to center and repeat to the other side. Do this 16 times (8 times on each side).

Too many people skip their stretches at the end of their workouts, and that's a shame. Although the studies about stretching's benefits have been contradictory in terms of injury prevention, its hard to ignore how relaxing it is. Also, I feel like it's the perfect way to switch from the energy of your workout to the rest of your day.

Side Leg Knee Bend and Leg Extension

100

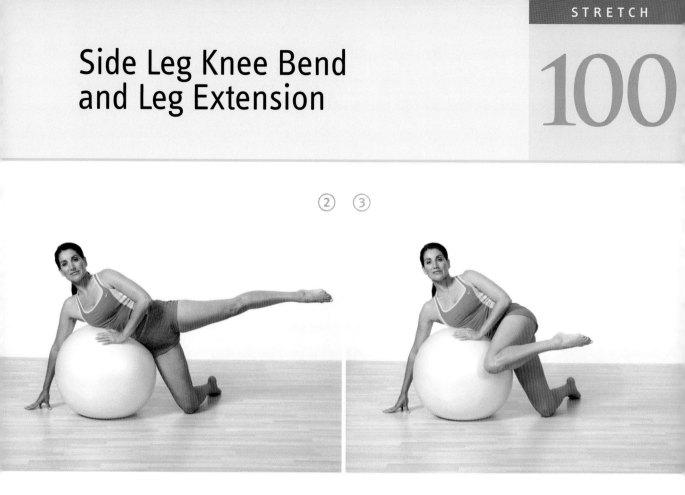

① Lie on your side with your torso draped over the ball, right hand on the floor, left hand on the ball. Your right knee should be bent, resting on the floor.

② Keeping your hips stacked, aligned, and steady using core strength, lift your left leg to hip height. This is your starting position.

③ Bring your left knee in toward your torso. You should feel a stretch in your gluteus maximus. Now, slowly bring your leg back out to the starting position with control. Repeat with your right leg.

101

Standing with Ball:
Calf Stretch with Balance

① ① Stand with feet close together, ball in front of your torso, body long. Raise the heel of your left foot, feeling the movement through your whole foot. Come down and repeat on the right foot.

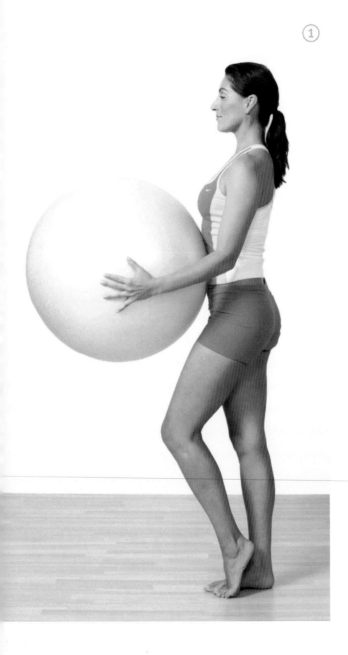

Thirty-Minute Workout

The key to a great thirty-minute workout is intensity. Most people think a shorter workout is easier than a longer workout, but that's not true. Most people—even the fittest athletes—can't do a high-intensity workout for a long time. So, if you're going to only exercise for a half hour, make it a worthwhile half hour.

In this workout, we don't move from floor to wall to floor again. We stay in one place in order to save time and keep our workout effective too. That's a good tip to keep in mind if you have five or ten minutes to spare. Decide how you're going to use the ball—against the wall, on the floor, or standing—and just do a little routine in that position.

Thirty-Minute Workout

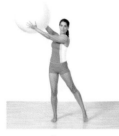

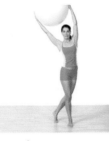

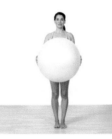

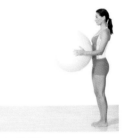

MOVE 5

Double Side Step with Ball Twist and Reach
(page 36)

Do this 16 times in each direction and go straight into the next move.

MOVE 6

Grapevine with Ball Overhead Circles
(page 37)

Do this 8 times in each direction and go straight into the next move.

MOVE 27

Walk in Place with Ball Held at Chest Level
(page 58)

Do this 32 times (16 times on each foot).

MOVE 13

March in Place with Ball Held at Chest Level
(page 44)

Do this 16 times (8 times with each foot).

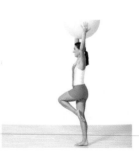

MOVE 14

March in Place with Ball Overhead Reaches
(page 45)

Do this 16 times (8 times with each foot).

Thirty-Minute Workout

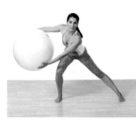

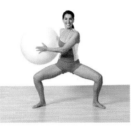

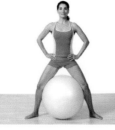

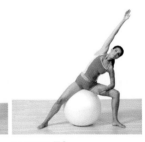

MOVE 20

Standing Side Lunges with Low Ball Reach
(page 51)

Do this 16 times (8 times on each side).

MOVE 19

Standing Pliés with Ball Side Twist
(page 50)

Do this 16 times (8 times on each side).

MOVE 16

Seated Pliés with Ball between Legs and Squeeze
(page 47)

Do this 16 times.

MOVE 70

Seated Side Lunges
(page 102)

Do this 16 times (8 times on each side).

POST CARDIO STRETCH

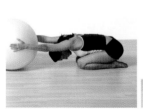

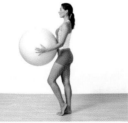

MOVE 94

On the Floor: Child's Pose
(page 127)

Hold this for 10 seconds (or longer) as you take deep breaths.

MOVE 101

Standing with Ball: Calf Stretch with Balance
(page 134)

Do this 16 times (8 times on each side).

Thirty-Minute Workout

TONING

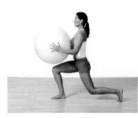 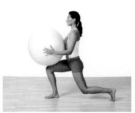 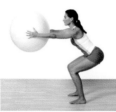 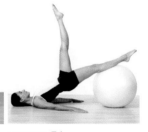

MOVE 72

Standing Front Lunge
(page 104)

Do this 8 times with your right leg forward, then switch legs and repeat.

MOVE 87

Walking Lunges
(page 119)

Do this 4 times forward, turn around, do it 4 times the other way, then repeat the sequence in both directions.

MOVE 73

Standing Squats Holding Ball
(page 105)

Do this quickly, one count as you come up, one count as you go down. Repeat 16 times.

MOVE 51

On the Floor: Pelvic Peel
(page 83)

Do this 8 times.

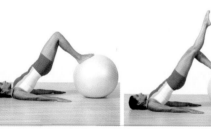

MOVE 49

On the Floor: Leg Pull Hamstring Curl
(page 81)

Do this 16 times.

MOVE 54

On the Floor: Single Leg Hamstring Curl
(page 86)

Do this 16 times (which will probably be hard at first). Switch sides.

Thirty-Minute Workout

THE MAMBO

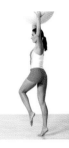 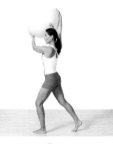 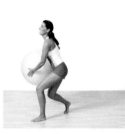 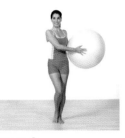

MOVE 3

Cross Step Walk Front with Ball Raise
(page 34)

Go forward 4 steps, then come back 4 steps. Do this 4 times in each direction, 16 times total.

MOVE 12

Mambo with Ball Twist
(page 43)

Do this 4 times then go directly into the next step.

MOVE 18

Sideways Mambo with Ball Raises
(page 49)

Do this 8 times on each side (in between you do the Cha-Cha to switch sides), then go immediately into the next step.

MOVE 2

Cha-Cha with Mambo
(page 33)

*Do this once on each side, then go right back into the **mambo**. Repeat this whole sequence 20 times. The Cha-Cha is your transition step to get from your right mambo to your left mambo—this is dancing!*

CARDIO COMBO

Put the above moves together, doing one after the other in one direction, then in the other direction. Do 4 times in each direction.

Thirty-Minute Workout

TONING AT THE WALL

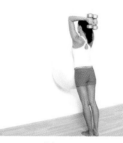

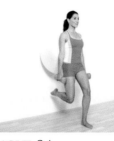

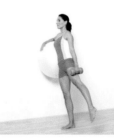

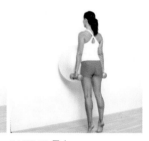

MOVE 81

Standing Wall Overhead Triceps Extensions with Dumbbells
(page 113)

Do two sets of 8.

MOVE 84

Standing Wall Single Leg Squat with Dumbbells
(page 116)

Come back to the start position and repeat the move 8 times. Do the exercise on the other side. This exercise can be very intense so start off slow and build up to more reps.

MOVE 75

Standing Wall Leg Lift Sides
(page 107)

Do this 16 times then switch sides.

MOVE 74

Standing Wall Calf Raises
(page 106)

Do this 16 times.

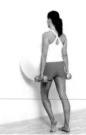

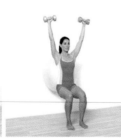

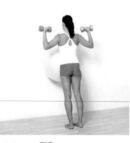

MOVE 82

Standing Wall Prances
(page 114)

Do this 32 times (16 times on each foot). You can do two sets if you want.

MOVE 80

Standing Wall Overhead Shoulder Press with Squat Holding Dumbbells
(page 112)

Do this 16 times.

MOVE 79

Standing Wall Overhead Shoulder Press with Calf Raises Dumbbells
(page 111)

Do this 16 times.

Thirty-Minute Workout

CARDIO SEQUENCE #3

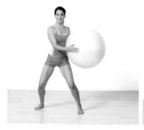

MOVE 23
Tap Side with Ball Twist
(page 54)

Try it in every direction 16 times.

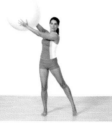

MOVE 5
Double Side Step with Ball Twist and Reach
(page 36)

Do this 16 times in each direction, going straight into the next move.

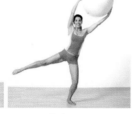

MOVE 24
Traveling Side Chasé with Ball Overhead Circles
(page 55)

*Do this 1 time to the right, then go into the **Tap Side with Ball Twist**. Do this 4 times. Now do the **Traveling Side Chasé with Ball Overhead Circles** once to the left. Repeat this whole series 4 times.*

Now put all of these cardio moves together into a combination, moving from the taps to the side steps to the traveling side chases and back to the side steps. Do your moves to the music and keep going for 3 minutes.

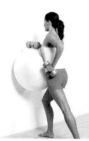

MOVE 78
Standing Wall Lunge Front: Single Arm Row with Dumbbells
(page 110)

Do this 16 times each side.

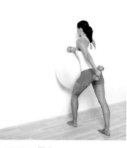

MOVE 76
Standing Wall Lunge Front: Triceps Kick-Back
(page 108)

Do this 16 times each side.

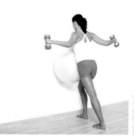

MOVE 77
Standing Wall Lunge Front: Reverse Fly with Dumbbells
(page 109)

Do this 16 times.

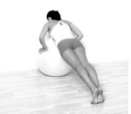

MOVE 83
Standing Wall Push-Ups
(page 115)

Do this 16 times.

Thirty-Minute Workout

FINAL STRETCH

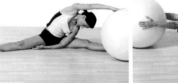 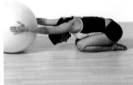

MOVE 95

On the Floor: Leg Straddle Wide Side Arm Reach
(page 128)

Hold this for 5 breath cycles (inhale and exhale is one cycle). Come back to start and repeat on the other side.

MOVE 94

On the Floor: Child's Pose
(page 127)

Hold this for 5 breath cycles (inhale and exhale is one cycle) and then come up to the start position. Repeat as often as you like.

Sixty-Minute Workout

Create some space in your living room or bedroom, turn on your iPod or burn a bouncy, energetic CD and get ready to move at an intense, fairly steady pace for one hour. Of course, you'll have to look at the book between each move to see what step comes next, but after a few times of doing the program, you'll get the hang of it and will probably only have to refer to the book every once in a while.

This isn't an easy workout and you should really keep moving in a big way. By big, I mean, make your movements large—reach high with the ball. If you are doing a squat, go low. The ball acts as resistance, but you still need to use your body effectively—so be strong and long.

Now, this is a sixty-minute routine, just like the kind you would find in a gym or an exercise studio. That means you need to go through the workout at a pretty good pace.

Sixty-Minute Workout

CARDIO COMBO #1

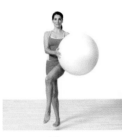

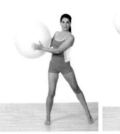

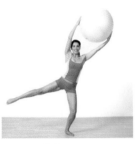

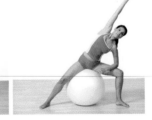

MOVE 15

**March in Place
with Ball Twist**
(page 46)

*Do this 16 times (8 times
on each foot).*

MOVE 21

**Step Touch
with Ball Twist**
(page 52)

*Do this 16 times (8 times
on each side).*

MOVE 4

**Double Side Step with
Ball Reach Side**
(page 35)

*Do this once to the right.
Then do 4 **March in
Place with Ball Twist**.
Another **Double Side
Step with Ball Reach
Side** to the left. Then do
4 **March in Place with
Ball Twist**. Repeat this
whole series 4 times.*

MOVE 24

**Traveling Side Chasé With
Ball Overhead Circles**
(page 55)

*Do this once to the right,
then go into the **Step
Touch with Ball Twist**.
Do this 4 times. Now do
the **Traveling Side
Chasé with Ball
Overhead Circles** once
to the left. Repeat this
whole series 4 times.*

CARDIO COOLDOWN

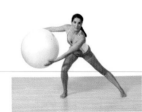

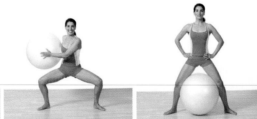

MOVE 20

**Standing Side Lunges
with Low Ball Reach**
(page 51)

*Do this 16 times (8 times
on each side).*

MOVE 19

**Standing Pliés
with Ball Side Twist**
(page 50)

*Do this 16 times (8 times
on each side).*

MOVE 16

**Seated Pliés with Ball
between Legs and
Squeeze**
(page 47)

Do this 16 times.

MOVE 91

Seated Side Lunges
(page 124)

*Do this 16 times (8 times
on each side).*

Sixty-Minute Workout

STRETCHES

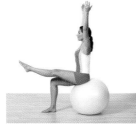

MOVE 67

Seated on Ball: Single Leg Extension
(page 99)

Do this 4 times, then go to the other side. Do another set on each side.

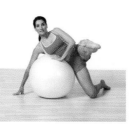

MOVE 93

Leaning on Ball: Side Leg Kick Front and Back
(page 126)

Do 2 sets.

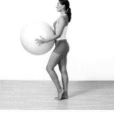

MOVE 101

Standing with Ball: Calf Stretch with Balance
(page 134)

Do this 16 times (8 times on each side).

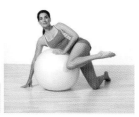

MOVE 100

Side Leg Knee Bend and Leg Extension
(page 133)

Hold this stretch for 20 seconds.

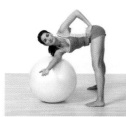

MOVE 92

Leaning on Ball: Shoulder Stretch
(page 125)

Hold this for 20 seconds, then repeat on the other side.

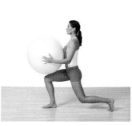

MOVE 71

Standing Back Lunge
(page 103)

Do this 8 times with your right foot, then switch to your left. Repeat the sequence one more time.

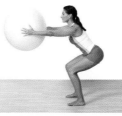

MOVE 73

Standing Squats Holding Ball
(page 105)

Do this 16 times.

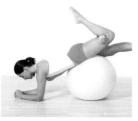

MOVE 39

Lay Over Ball: Hamstring Curl with Dumbbells
(page 71)

Do this 16 times (8 times on each side).

STRETCHES CONTINUED ON NEXT PAGE

Sixty-Minute Workout

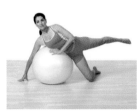 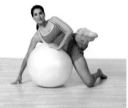 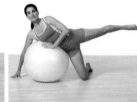

MOVE 93

Leaning on Ball: Side Leg Kick Front and Back
(page 126)

Repeat the sequence 16 times. Then repeat on the other side.

MOVE 70

Leaning on Ball: Front Leg Lift Pulses
(page 102)

Do this 16 times (8 times on each side).

MOVE 56

Leaning on Ball: Back Leg Lift Pulses
(page 88)

Do this 16 times (8 times on each side).

CARDIO COMBO #2

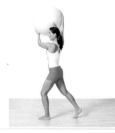 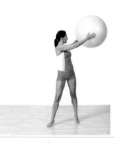 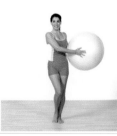 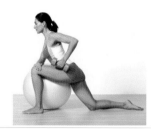

MOVE 12

Mambo with Ball Twist
(page 43)

Do this 4 times then go directly into the next step.

MOVE 18

Sideways Mambo with Ball Raises
(page 49)

Do this 8 times on each side (in between you do the Cha-Cha to switch sides), then go immediately into the next step.

MOVE 2

Cha-Cha with Mambo
(page 33)

*Do this once on each side, then go right back into the **Mambo**. Repeat this whole sequence 20 times. The Cha-Cha is your transition step to get from your right mambo to your left mambo.*

MOVE 30

Kneeling Over Ball: Single Arm Row with Dumbbells
(page 62)

Do this 16 times, then switch sides.

Sixty-Minute Workout

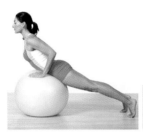

MOVE 7

Kneeling Over Ball: Lean Away with Elbows
(page 38)

Hold this for 5 breath cycles (inhale and exhale is one cycle). Then come down. Repeat as many times as you like, focusing on the length of your spine each time.

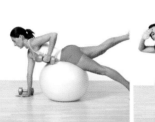

MOVE 40

Lay Chest Over Ball: Lat Pull with Leg Extension
(page 72)

Do this 16 times. Repeat on the other side.

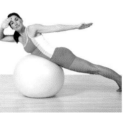

MOVE 11

Lay Chest Over Ball: Back Extension with Oblique Twist
(page 42)

Do 16 on each side.

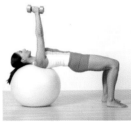

MOVE 36

Lay Back Over Ball: Pull over with Dumbbells
(page 68)

Do this 16 times.

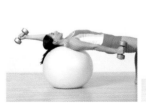

MOVE 35

Lay Back Over Ball: The Go-Go with Dumbbells
(page 67)

Do this 16 times.

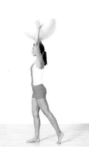

MOVE 26

Walk Front/Back with Ball Overhead Reach
(page 57)

Do this 8 steps forward, then 8 steps back.

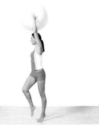

MOVE 3

Cross Step Walk Front with Ball Raise
(page 34)

Go forward 4 steps, then come back 4 steps. Do this 4 times in each direction, 16 times total.

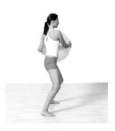

MOVE 23

Tap Side with Ball Twist
(page 54)

Do this in every direction 16 times.

CARDIO COMBO #2 CONTINUED ON NEXT PAGE

Sixty-Minute Workout

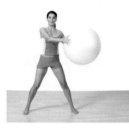

MOVE 22

**Tap Side with
a Twist and Turn**

(page 53)

*Do this 8 times to each
side.*

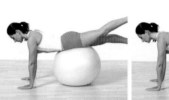

MOVE 9

**Lay Over Ball:
Leg Lift Circle**

(page 40)

*Do this 8 times, then
repeat on the other side.*

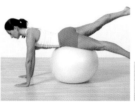

MOVE 38

**Lay Over Ball:
Flutter Kick**

(page 70)

Do this 16 times.

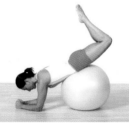

MOVE 8

**Lay Over Ball:
The Double Leg Lift**

(page 39)

*Do this 8 times. Rest a
minute (you can relax
over the ball if you want)
and then do 8 more times.*

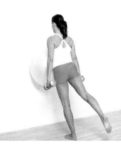

MOVE 85

**Standing Wall
Leg Lift Rear**

(page 117)

*Do this 16 times.
Switch legs.*

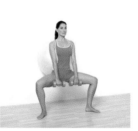

MOVE 86

**Standing Wall Pliés
with Dumbbells**

(page 118)

Do this 16 times.

Sixty-Minute Workout

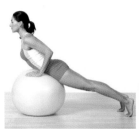

MOVE 7

Kneeling Over Ball: Lean Away with Elbows
(page 38)

Hold this for 5 breath cycles (inhale and exhale is one cycle). Then come down. Repeat as many times as you like, focusing on the length of your spine each time.

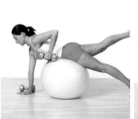

MOVE 40

Lay Chest Over Ball: Lat Pull with Leg Extension
(page 72)

Do this 16 times. Repeat on the other side.

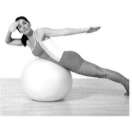

MOVE 11

Lay Chest Over Ball: Back Extension with Oblique Twist
(page 42)

Do 16 on each side.

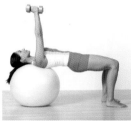

MOVE 36

Lay Back Over Ball: Pull over with Dumbbells
(page 68)

Do this 16 times.

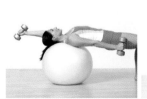

MOVE 35

Lay Back Over Ball: The Go-Go with Dumbbells
(page 67)

Do this 16 times.

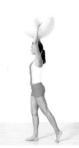

MOVE 26

Walk Front/Back with Ball Overhead Reach
(page 57)

Do this 8 steps forward, then 8 steps back.

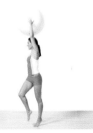

MOVE 3

Cross Step Walk Front with Ball Raise
(page 34)

Go forward 4 steps, then come back 4 steps. Do this 4 times in each direction, 16 times total.

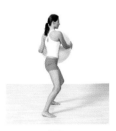

MOVE 23

Tap Side with Ball Twist
(page 54)

Do this in every direction 16 times.

CARDIO COMBO #2 CONTINUED ON NEXT PAGE

Sixty-Minute Workout

CARDIO COMBO #2 (CONT.)

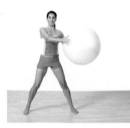

MOVE 22

**Tap Side with
a Twist and Turn**
(page 53)

*Do this 8 times to each
side.*

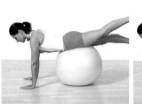

MOVE 9

**Lay Over Ball:
Leg Lift Circle**
(page 40)

*Do this 8 times, then
repeat on the other side.*

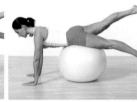

MOVE 38

**Lay Over Ball:
Flutter Kick**
(page 70)

Do this 16 times.

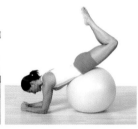

MOVE 8

**Lay Over Ball:
The Double Leg Lift**
(page 39)

*Do this 8 times. Rest a
minute (you can relax
over the ball if you want)
and then do 8 more times.*

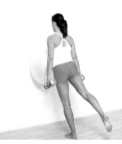

MOVE 85

**Standing Wall
Leg Lift Rear**
(page 117)

*Do this 16 times.
Switch legs.*

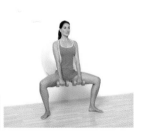

MOVE 86

**Standing Wall Pliés
with Dumbbells**
(page 118)

Do this 16 times.

Sixty-Minute Workout

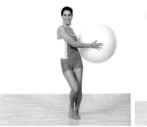

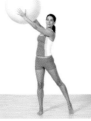

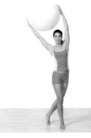

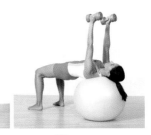

MOVE 21
Step Touch with Ball Twist
(page 52)

Do this 16 times (8 times on each side).

MOVE 4
Double Side Step with Ball Reach Side
(page 35)

*Do this once to the right. Then do 4 **Step Touch with Ball Twist**. Follow this with another **Double Side Step with Ball Reach Side** to the left. Then do 4 **Step Touch with Ball Twist**. Repeat this whole series 4 times.*

MOVE 6
Grapevine with Ball Overhead Circles
(page 37)

Do this 8 times in each direction.

MOVE 32
Lay Back Over Ball: Chest Fly with Dumbbells
(page 64)

Repeat 16 times.

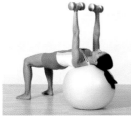

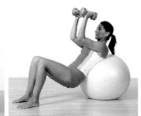

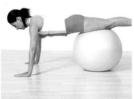

MOVE 33
Lay Back Over Ball: Chest Press with Dumbbells
(page 65)

Do this 16 times.

MOVE 28
Incline Chest Squeeze
(page 60)

Do this 16 times.

MOVE 41
Lay Chest Over Ball: Push-Ups
(page 73)

Do this up to 16 times (you might have to work up to this number).

Sixty-Minute Workout

UPPER BODY TONING

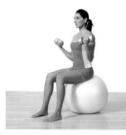 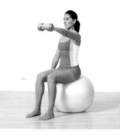 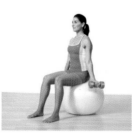 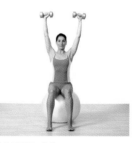

MOVE 66

Seated on Ball: The Sevens
(page 98)

Do this 16 times.

MOVE 62

Seated on Ball: Front Arm Raises with Dumbbells
(page 94)

Do 16 times on each side.

MOVE 69

Seated on Ball: Side Sevens
(page 101)

Do 16 times on each side.

MOVE 64

Seated on Ball: Overhead Shoulder Press with Dumbbells
(page 96)

Do this 16 times.

CARDIO COMBO #1

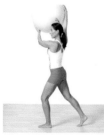 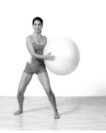 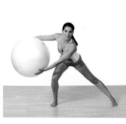 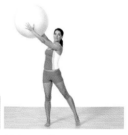

MOVE 12

Mambo with Ball Twist
(page 43)

Do this 4 times then go directly into the next step.

MOVE 23

Tap Side with Ball Twist
(page 54)

Do this in every direction 16 times.

MOVE 20

Standing Side Lunges with Low Ball Reach
(page 51)

Do this 16 times (8 times on each side).

MOVE 4

Double Side Step with Ball Reach Side
(page 35)

*Do this once to the right. Then do 4 **Tap Side with Ball Twist**. Follow this with another **Double Side Step with Ball Reach Side** to the left. Then do 4 **Tap Side with Ball Twist**. Repeat this whole series 4 times.*

Sixty-Minute Workout

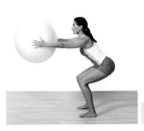

MOVE 73

Standing Squats Holding Ball
(page 105)

Do this 16 times.

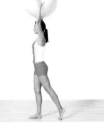

MOVE 26

Walk Front/Back with Ball Overhead Reach
(page 57)

Do this 16 times (8 times in each direction).

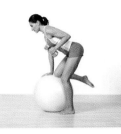

MOVE 31

Kneeling on Ball: Triceps Extension
(page 63)

Do this 8 times. Rest for ten seconds, then do 8 more times.

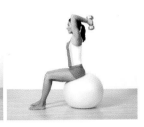

MOVE 68

Seated on Ball: Triceps Overhead Extension with Dumbbells
(page 100)

Do two sets of 8 reps.

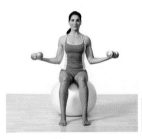

MOVE 65

Seated on Ball: Rotator Cuff
(page 97)

Do this 16 times.

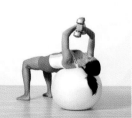

MOVE 34

Lay Back Over Ball: Cross Triceps Extensions with Dumbbells
(page 66)

Return to the start and repeat 16 times.

Sixty-Minute Workout

BODY TONING: ABS

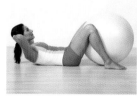

MOVE 46

On the Floor: Inner Thigh Squeeze with Abdominal Curl
(page 78)

Do this 16 times.

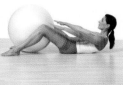

MOVE 48

On the Floor: Inner Thigh Squeeze with Roll Up
(page 80)

Do this 8 times (if you can). Do another 8 reps.

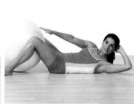

MOVE 47

On the Floor: Inner Thigh Squeeze with Oblique Arm Reach
(page 79)

Do this 16 times. Repeat on the other side.

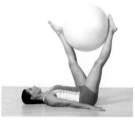

MOVE 53

On the Floor: Scissors Twist with Legs
(page 85)

Do this 32 times (16 times in each direction).

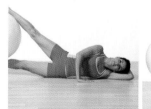

MOVE 44

On the Floor: Double Leg Lift Side with Inner Thigh Squeeze
(page 76)

Do this 16 times, then switch sides. An added bonus: If you try lifting your bottom side's waistline off the floor, you'll tone both sides of your obliques during this move!

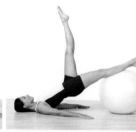

MOVE 52

On the Floor: The Roll Over
(page 84)

Do this 3 times.

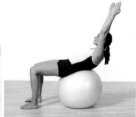

MOVE 51

On the Floor: Pelvic Peel
(page 83)

Do this 32 times (16 times on each side).

MOVE 58

Seated on Ball: Abdominal Curl with Arm Reach
(page 90)

Do this 16 times.

Sixty-Minute Workout

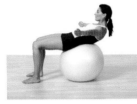

MOVE 57

**Seated on Ball:
Abdominal Curl
with Arm Circles**
(page 89)

Do this 16 times.

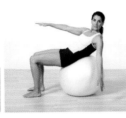

MOVE 59

**Seated on Ball:
Abdominal Curl with
Single Arm Reach Back**
(page 91)

Do this 16 times.

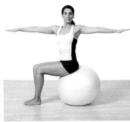

MOVE 61

**Seated on Ball:
Core Twist**
(page 93)

*Do this 16 times (8 times
on each side).*

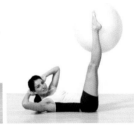

MOVE 50

**On the Floor:
Oblique Twist**
(page 82)

*Do this 32 times (16 times
on each side).*

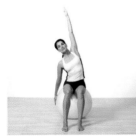

MOVE 99

**Seated on Ball:
Side Stretch**
(page 132)

*Do this 16 times (8 times
on each side).*

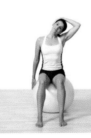

MOVE 97

**Seated on Ball:
Neck Stretch**
(page 130)

*Hold this for 10 seconds
and then repeat on the
other side. You can do this
twice if you want.*

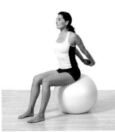

MOVE 96

**Seated on Ball:
Chest Stretch**
(page 129)

*Hold this for as long as
you like (at least 30 second) to feel the stretch in
your back.*

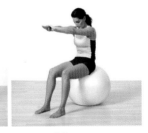

MOVE 98

**Seated on Ball:
Rhomboid Stretch**
(page 131)

Hold this for 10 seconds.

BODY TONING: ABS CONTINUED ON NEXT PAGE

Sixty-Minute Workout

BODY TONING: ABS (CONT.)

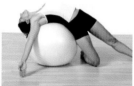 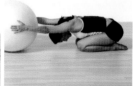

MOVE 89

**Lay Back Over Ball:
Open Chest Stretch**
(page 122)

*Hold this for 30 seconds,
then switch sides. You can
do this twice if you want.*

MOVE 94

On the Floor: Child's Pose
(page 127)

*Hold this for 30 seconds
(or longer) as you take
deep breaths.*

Ten Specialized Workouts

Nothing can really replace a full-blown workout. Keeping your heart rate up and your muscles moving is the true way to fitness. However, I believe—and studies have shown—that shorter workouts and shorter bouts of movement are important to both health and fitness. Sitting in front of a TV for hours on end, sitting in a car, sitting at a desk…well, you see the problem. It's just impossible to burn calories and keep your heart in shape if you're sitting all the time.

Of course, it's difficult in this day and age to not sit a lot, but this chapter will help you incorporate shorter workouts into your life. Don't discount the benefits of a five-minute abs program or a twenty-minute exercise program. Five minutes is plenty of time to work most muscles groups and a high-intensity twenty-minute program will keep your heart rate up at a higher level than a sixty-minute class will. These shorter programs are a perfect complement to your longer weekly or twice-weekly workouts.

Twenty-Minute Full Body Program

This routine is the perfect combination of cardio, upper body, lower body, and core moves. In it, you'll do each move for one minute so your heart rate will stay up the entire twenty minutes, even while you're strength training. And your whole body will get a full-body strengthening workout, too!

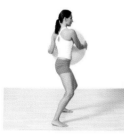

MOVE 23

Tap Side with Ball Twist
(page 54)

Do this for a full minute

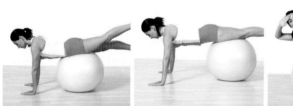

MOVE 9

Lay Over Ball: Leg Lift Circle
(page 40)

Do this at least 16 times, then switch legs. Do this for one minute.

MOVE 41

Lay Chest Over Ball: Push-Ups
(page 73)

Do this 16 times (you might have to work up to this number).

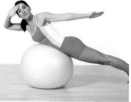

MOVE 11

Lay Chest Over Ball: Back Extension with Oblique Twist
(page 42)

Do 16 on each side.

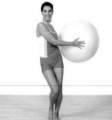

MOVE 17

Side Step "Step Touch" with Ball Twist
(page 48)

Do this for one minute.

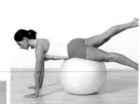

MOVE 38

Lay Over Ball: Flutter Kick
(page 70)

Do this for the entire minute.

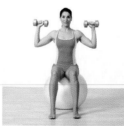

MOVE 64

Seated on Ball: Overhead Shoulder Press with Dumbbells
(page 96)

Do this 16 times.

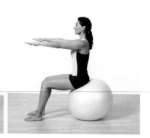

MOVE 60

Seated on Ball: Abdominal Curl-Up
(page 92)

Do this for one minute.

Twenty-Minute Full Body Program

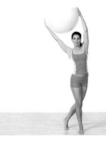

MOVE 6

Grapevine with Ball Overhead Circles
(page 37)

Do this in each direction for the entire minute.

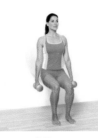

MOVE 88

Wall Squat
(page 120)

Do this for one minute.

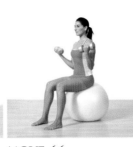

MOVE 66

Seated on Ball: The Sevens
(page 98)

Do this 16 times in each direction.

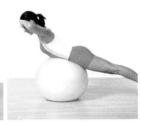

MOVE 10

Lay Chest Over Ball: Back Extension
(page 41)

Do this 16 times.

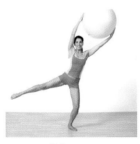

MOVE 24

Traveling Side Chasé With Ball Overhead Circles
(page 55)

Do this from side to side for the full minute.

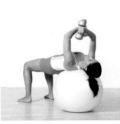

MOVE 74

Standing Wall Calf Raises
(page 106)

Do this slowly for the full minute.

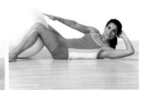

MOVE 34

Lay Back over Ball: Cross Triceps Extensions with Dumbbells
(page 66)

Do this for one minute.

MOVE 47

On the Floor: Inner Thigh Squeeze with Oblique Arm Reach
(page 79)

Do this 32 times (16 times on each side). This should take a full minute.

Twenty-Minute Full Body Program

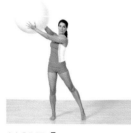

MOVE 5

Double Side Step with Ball Twist and Reach
(page 36)

Do this in each direction for the full minute.

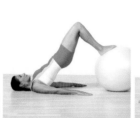

MOVE 49

On the Floor: Leg Pull Hamstring Curl
(page 81)

Do this slowly for the full minute.

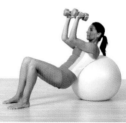

MOVE 28

Incline Chest Squeeze
(page 60)

Do this for one minute.

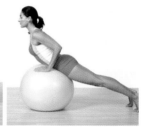

MOVE 7

Kneeling Over Ball: Lean Away with Elbows
(page 38)

Hold this for 5 breath cycles (inhale and exhale is one cycle). Then come down. Repeat as many times as you like, focusing on the length of your spine each time.

Fifteen-Minute
Full Body Program

The secret to this program is to move quickly and not take any time to rest. You'll only do one set of every move so your heart rate will stay up.

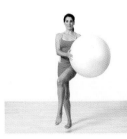

MOVE 15

**March in Place
with Ball Twist**
(page 46)

*Do this 16 times (8 times
on each foot).*

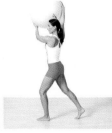

MOVE 12

Mambo with Ball Twist
(page 43)

*Do this 4 times then go
directly into the next step.*

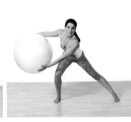

MOVE 20

**Standing Side Lunges
with Low Ball Reach**
(page 51)

*Do this 16 times (8 times
on each side).*

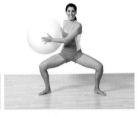

MOVE 19

**Standing Pliés
with Ball Side Twist**
(page 50)

*Do this 16 times (8 times
on each side).*

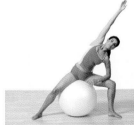

MOVE 91

Seated Side Lunges
(page 124)

*Do this 16 times (8 times
on each side).*

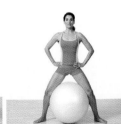

MOVE 16

**Seated Pliés with Ball
between Legs and
Squeeze**
(page 47)

Do this 16 times.

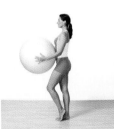

MOVE 101

**Standing with Ball: Calf
Stretch with Balance**
(page 134)

*Do this 16 times (8 times
on each side).*

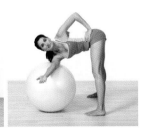

MOVE 92

**Leaning on Ball:
Shoulder Stretch**
(page 125)

*Hold this for 30 seconds,
then switch to the other
side.*

Fifteen-Minute Full Body Program

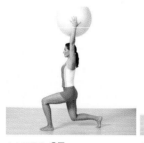

MOVE 87

Walking Lunges
(page 119)

Do this 4 times forward, turn around, do it 4 times the other way, then repeat the sequence in both directions.

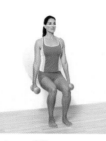

MOVE 88

Wall Squat
(page 120)

Do this 16 times.

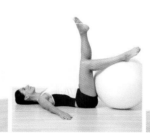

MOVE 45

On the Floor: Hip Rolls with Leg Extension
(page 77)

Do this 16 times (8 times on each side).

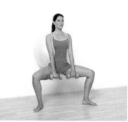

MOVE 86

Standing Wall Pliés with Dumbbells
(page 118)

Do this 16 times.

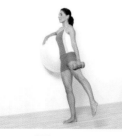

MOVE 75

Standing Wall Leg Lift Sides
(page 107)

Do this 16 times, then switch sides.

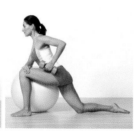

MOVE 30

Kneeling Over Ball: Single Arm Row with Dumbbells
(page 62)

Do this 16 times, then switch sides.

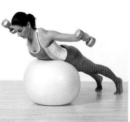

MOVE 29

Kneeling Over Ball: Reverse Fly with Dumbbells
(page 61)

Do this 16 times slowly.

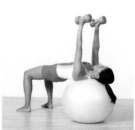
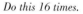

MOVE 32

Lay Back Over Ball: Chest Fly with Dumbbells
(page 64)

Do this 16 times.

Fifteen-Minute
Full Body Program

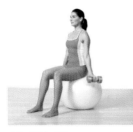

MOVE 69

**Seated on Ball:
Side Sevens**
(page 101)

*Do this 16 times (8 times
on each side).*

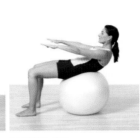

MOVE 60

**Seated on Ball:
Abdominal Curl-Up**
(page 92)

*Come back down slowly
and repeat 16 times.*

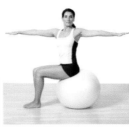

MOVE 61

**Seated on Ball:
Core Twist**
(page 93)

*Do this 16 times (8 times
on each side).*

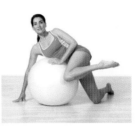

MOVE 100

**Side Leg Knee Bend
and Leg Extension**
(page 133)

*Do this 16 times (8 times
on each side).*

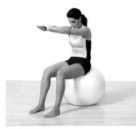

MOVE 98

**Seated on Ball:
Rhomboid Stretch**
(page 131)

Hold this for 10 seconds.

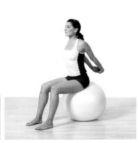

MOVE 96

**Seated on Ball: Chest
Stretch**
(page 129)

*Hold this for as long as
you like (at least 30 second) to feel the stretch in
your back.*

Ten-Minute
Full Body Program

Ten minutes is a down-and-dirty, get-your-endorphins-up-and-your-body-moving routine. You won't focus on any one body part or burn a lot of calories, but if you've been sitting a long time, taking a ten-minute break will really help your body relax and get re-energized.

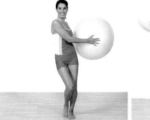

MOVE 17

Side Step "Step Touch" with Ball Twist
(page 48)

Do this 16 times in each direction.

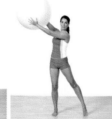

MOVE 5

Double Side Step with Ball Twist and Reach
(page 36)

Do this 16 times in each direction, going straight into the next move.

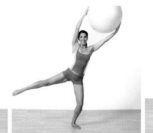

MOVE 24

Traveling Side Chasé with Ball Overhead Circles
(page 55)

Do this 16 times (8 times on each side).

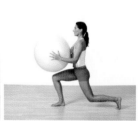

MOVE 72

Standing Front Lunge
(page 104)

Do this 8 times with your right leg forward, then switch legs. Repeat on each side.

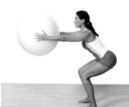

MOVE 73

Standing Squats Holding Ball
(page 105)

Do this 16 times.

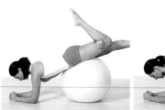

MOVE 39

Lay Over Ball: Hamstring Curl with Dumbbell
(page 71)

Do this 16 times, then switch to the other side.

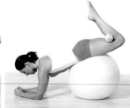

MOVE 37

Lay Over Ball: Double Leg Hamstring Curl with Dumbbell
(page 69)

Do this 16 times.

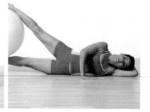

MOVE 44

On the Floor: Double Leg Lift Side with Inner Thigh Squeeze
(page 76)

Do this 16 times, then switch to the other side.

Ten-Minute Full Body Program

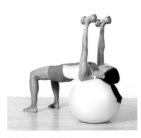

MOVE 32

Lay Back Over Ball: Chest Fly with Dumbbells
(page 64)

Do this 16 times.

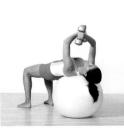

MOVE 34

Lay Back Over Ball: Cross Triceps Extensions with Dumbbells
(page 66)

Do this 16 times.

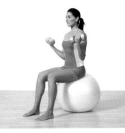

MOVE 66

Seated on Ball: The Sevens
(page 98)

Do this 16 times.

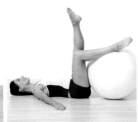

MOVE 45

On the Floor: Hip Rolls with Leg Extension
(page 77)

Do this 16 times (8 times to each side).

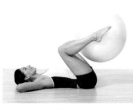

MOVE 42

On the Floor: Abdominal Curl with Leg Extension
(page 74)

Do this 16 times. Do 2 sets.

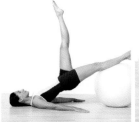

MOVE 51

On the Floor: Pelvic Peel
(page 83)

Do this 32 times (16 times on each side).

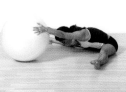

MOVE 90

On the Floor: Straddle Stretch to the Side
(page 123)

Hold this for 5 breath cycles (inhale and exhale is one cycle). Come back to start and repeat on the other side.

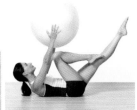

MOVE 55

On the Floor: Single Leg Stretch
(page 87)

Do this 16 times (8 times on each leg).

Ten-Minute Full Body Program

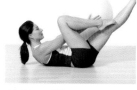

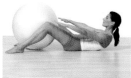

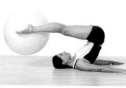

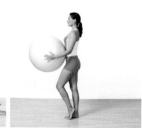

MOVE 43

On the Floor: Crisscross
(page 75)

Do this 16 times (8 times on each leg).

MOVE 48

On the Floor: Inner Thigh Squeeze with Roll Up
(page 80)

Do this 16 times (if you can).

MOVE 52

On the Floor: The Roll Over
(page 84)

Do this 3 times.

MOVE 101

Standing with Ball: Calf Stretch with Balance
(page 134)

Do this 16 times (8 times on each side).

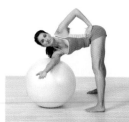

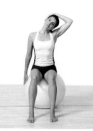

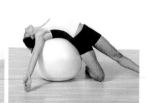

MOVE 92

Leaning on Ball: Shoulder Stretch
(page 125)

Hold this for 20 seconds, then go to the other side.

MOVE 97

Seated on Ball: Neck Stretch
(page 130)

Hold this for 10 seconds and then repeat on the other side. You can do this twice if you want.

MOVE 89

Lay Back Over Ball: Open Chest Stretch
(page 122)

Hold this for 10 seconds, then switch sides. You can do this twice if you want.

Five-Minute Abs

The secret to this routine is that you're going to do each exercise twice for maximum muscle burn. Don't rush through it and remember to breathe properly—exhale on the effort (lifting up) and inhale as you release (lower your torso).

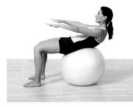

MOVE 60

Seated on Ball: Abdominal Curl-Up
(page 92)

Do this 16 times.

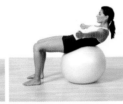

MOVE 57

Seated on Ball: Abdominal Curl with Arm Circles
(page 89)

Do this 16 times.

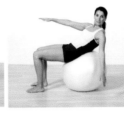

MOVE 59

Seated on Ball: Abdominal Curl with Single Arm Reach Back
(page 91)

Do this 16 times.

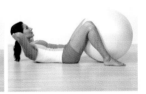

MOVE 46

On the Floor: Inner Thigh Squeeze with Abdominal Curl
(page 78)

Do this 16 times.

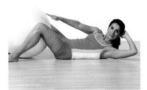

MOVE 47

On the Floor: Inner Thigh Squeeze with Oblique Arm Reach
(page 79)

Do this 32 times (16 times on each side).

Now go back to the start and do the whole routine one more time.

Five-Minute Legs

If you really want a perfect leg workout, combine this routine with a walk, which not only trims your legs, but also burns off fat. And if you want to do some butt-sculpting, walk up some hills. Then you'll really see a difference in your lower body.

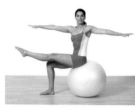 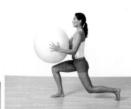 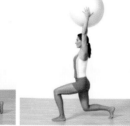 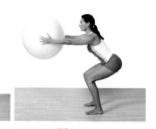

MOVE 67

Seated on Ball: Single Leg Extension
(page 99)

Do this 16 times on each side.

MOVE 72

Standing Front Lunge
(page 104)

Do this 8 times with your right leg forward, then switch legs. Repeat on each side.

MOVE 87

Walking Lunges
(page 119)

Do this 4 times forward, turn around, do it 4 times the other way, then repeat the sequence in both directions.

MOVE 73

Standing Squats Holding Ball
(page 105)

Do this 16 times.

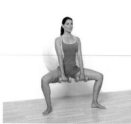 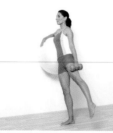 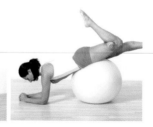

MOVE 86

Standing Wall Pliés with Dumbbells
(page 118)

Repeat 16 times.

MOVE 75

Standing Wall Leg Lift Sides
(page 107)

Do this 16 times, then switch sides.

MOVE 39

Lay Over Ball: Hamstring Curl with Dumbbell
(page 71)

Do this 16 times then switch sides.

Five-Minute Butt

A good butt has two things—a little bit of muscle and a little bit of fat. The muscle keeps your butt high and tight while the fat gives it some shape. Now, I realize a perfect butt isn't the most important thing in the world, but it is a sign that you are in pretty good health—because you can't sit too much and not exercise and have a nicely shaped rear. A good butt is a sign that you take care of yourself and are active.

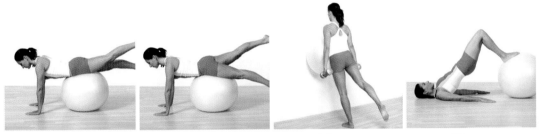

MOVE 9
Lay Over Ball:
Leg Lift Circle
(page 40)

Do this 16 times in each direction then switch legs.

MOVE 38
Lay Over Ball:
Flutter Kick
(page 70)

Do this 8 times then repeat on the other side.

MOVE 85
Standing Wall
Leg Lift Rear
(page 117)

Do this 8 times, then switch legs.

MOVE 49
On the Floor: Leg Pull
Hamstring Curl
(page 81)

Do this 16 times.

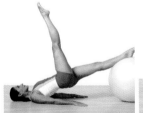

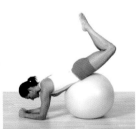

MOVE 54
On the Floor: Single Leg
Hamstring Curl
(page 86)

Do this 16 times (which will probably be hard at first). Switch sides.

MOVE 8
Lay Over Ball:
The Double Leg Lift
(page 39)

Do this 8 times. Rest a moment (you can relax over the ball if you want) and then do another 8.

Five-Minute Back

I can always tell when I haven't been taking care of myself because I slouch when I'm tired. Even though a strong, healthy back isn't the most eye-catching body part, it is very important and most fitness experts spend a lot of time strengthening their back muscles, because they know there is no way to hide a weak one. Standing tall and not having any aches or pains are the benefits of back exercises.

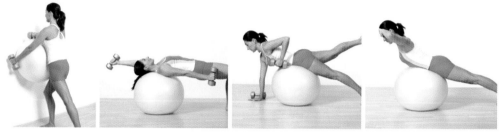

MOVE 78

Standing Wall Lunge Front: Single Arm Row with Dumbbells
(page 110)

Do this 16 times, then switch sides.

MOVE 35

Lay Back Over Ball: The Go-Go with Dumbbells
(page 67)

Do this 16 times.

MOVE 40

Lay Chest Over Ball: Lat Pull with Leg Extension
(page 72)

Do this 16 times, then switch sides.

MOVE 10

Lay Chest Over Ball: Back Extension
(page 41)

Do this 16 times.

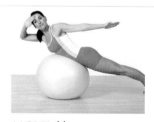

MOVE 11

Lay Chest Over Ball: Back Extension with Oblique Twist
(page 42)

Do this 16 times, then switch sides.

Five-Minute Arms

Sleeveless. How great is it to wear tank tops or camisoles or a pretty strapless dress? It really doesn't take that much to keep your arms in shape. Do this routine a few times a week and you'll see a real difference in the shape of your upper arms. And don't be afraid to use heavy weights—those women you see with the sleek arms probably lift heavier weights than you ever will.

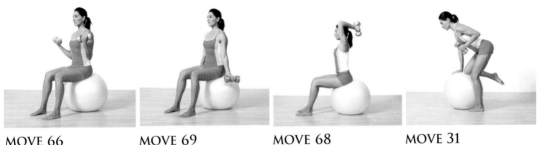

MOVE 66

**Seated on Ball:
The Sevens**
(page 98)

Do this 8 times for 2 sets.

MOVE 69

**Seated on Ball:
Side Sevens**
(page 101)

Do this 8 times for 2 sets.

MOVE 68

**Seated on Ball: Triceps
Overhead Extension with
Dumbbells**
(page 100)

Do this 8 times for 2 sets.

MOVE 31

**Kneeling on Ball:
Triceps Extension**
(page 63)

*Do this 8 times. Rest
for ten seconds, then do
8 more times.*

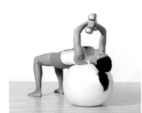

MOVE 34

**Lay Back Over Ball: Cross
Triceps Extensions with
Dumbbells**
(page 66)

Do this 16 times.

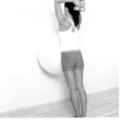

MOVE 81

**Standing Wall Overhead
Triceps Extensions with
Dumbbells**
(page 113)

Do two sets of 8 reps each.

Five-Minute Shoulders

One of my favorite body parts is the back of the shoulders, because when a woman is in shape, they get this lovely line from their back to their arm that just looks so elegant when it moves. A shapely shoulder is really muscular and sleek. You don't need heavy weights to change the way your shoulder looks, but you do need to work all three aspects of the muscle: front, middle, and back.

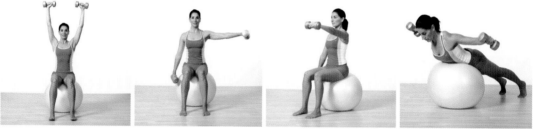

MOVE 64

Seated on Ball: Overhead Shoulder Press with Dumbbells (page 96)

Do this 16 times.

MOVE 63

Seated on Ball: Lateral Arm Raises with Dumbbells (page 95)

Do this 32 times (16 times on each side).

MOVE 62

Seated on Ball: Front Arm Raises with Dumbbells (page 94)

Do 16 times on each side.

MOVE 29

Kneeling Over Ball: Reverse Fly with Dumbbells (page 61)

Do this 16 times slowly.

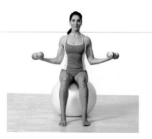

MOVE 65

Seated on Ball: Rotator Cuff (page 97)

Do this 16 times.

Five-Minute Pilates

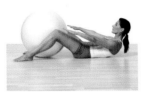

MOVE 48

On the Floor: Inner Thigh Squeeze with Roll Up
(page 80)

Do this 16 times (if you can).

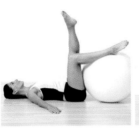

MOVE 45

On the Floor: Hip Rolls with Leg Extension
(page 77)

Do this 16 times (8 times to each side).

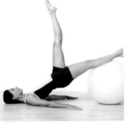

MOVE 51

On the Floor: Pelvic Peel
(page 83)

Do this 32 times (16 times on each side).

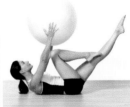

MOVE 55

On the Floor: Single Leg Stretch
(page 87)

Do this 16 times (8 times on each side).

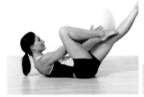

MOVE 43

On the Floor: Crisscross
(page 75)

Do this 16 times (8 times on each side).

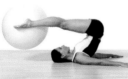

MOVE 52

On the Floor: The Roll Over
(page 84)

Do this 3 times.

Ball Glossary

Apex: The very top of the ball.

Atherosclerosis: Occurs when fat accumulates in the lining at the arterial wall, making blood vessels thinner and forcing the heart to work harder than usual to pump blood.

Core: The muscles of your trunk, including your spine, upper back, lower back, chest, and abdominals.

Deltoid: A shoulder muscle composed of three parts—the anterior, posterior, and medial.

Eractor spinae: A back muscle with the primary responsibility of extending the spine.

Gluteal muscles: The muscles on a person's rear end, which are composed of three parts—the gluteus maximus, gluteus medius, and gluteus minimus.

Internal and external oblique muscles: The abdominal muscles that allow you to twist and bend at the waist.

Latissimus dorsi: The latissimus dorsi are large muscles that wrap around your back.

Multifidus: A long and deep abdominal muscle. It's primary duty is to stabilize the spine and assist with extension (arching) and rotation (twisting).

Physiotherapy: Physical therapy programs to help injured people gain strength and to stabilize their muscles.

Port de bras: Means "carriage of the arms" in French, and describes the technique and practice of arm movement in ballet.

Pulse: Similar to a gentle bounce, you can pulse your body as you stretch without forcing any movement.

Sacrum: The last bone of the spine. The part of the vertebral column that directly connects with—and forms a part of—the pelvis.

Transversus abdominis: The deepest abdominal muscle, which wraps all the way around the waist .

Acknowledgments

To my students and clients for the years of support and loyalty that have enabled me to realize my dreams of owning my own business, starring in my own exercise videos, and publishing my first fitness book. I am grateful for the honest feedback from my group exercise class over the past fifteen years.

To the teachers who have inspired me to perfect my teaching skills and to lead by example. My master instructor, Real Isaeowitz, is one of the greatest instructors I have trained with. The same goes with Elizabeth Larkam, Lolita San Miguel, Allan Herdman, Madeline Black, Kathy Murakami, Debbie and Carlos Rosas, and Bruno Bosardi.

To Angie Bunch, who lead me into my career path of fitness. To my first dance teacher, Miss Eva. Thank you.

To my girlfriends who add sunshine to my life: Portia Page, Wendy Szoke, Michelle Morgan, Dion Kentner, Lisa Moore, Amber Brown, Andrea Davis, Christina Carreno, Sheri Laine, Trina Johnson, Gaynor Dalbrat, Deborah McCloud, Aubri Almendariz, Carrie Weilan, Dana Race, Micki Papini, Pamela Barnhart.

To the women I admire: Melissa McNeese, Donna Raskin, Andrea Ambandos—Yes, you did discover me!—Sabine Anderson, Tamilee Webb, Debbie Rosas, Gloria Gonzales, Debbie Ford, and Oprah Winfrey. These women have it all—leadership, determination, and passion.

And lastly…

To my husband Pete Tillack: without your daily cooking and cleaning this book would have not been finished. Stinky, I love you.

About the Author

Lizbeth Garcia, owner of Tilcia Studios in La Jolla, California, has been a fitness instructor in San Diego for fifteen years. A certified Pilates trainer, she has been featured in many publications, including *Shape*, *Fitness*, and *Health Magazine*, which named her *On the Ball Pilates Workout for Beginners* video the best Pilates video of the year in 2005. For more information, visit www.LizbethGarica.com. Lizbeth lives in Southern California.

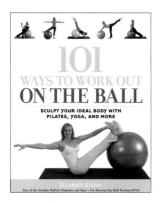

101 WAYS TO WORK OUT ON THE BALL
by Elizabeth Gillies
ISBN: 1-59233-084-3
$19.95
Paperback; 176 pages
Available wherever books are sold

SCULPT YOUR IDEAL BODY WITH PILATES, YOGA, AND MORE

Everyone loves the workout ball! It can help with weight training, Pilates, yoga, and even cardio and stretching moves. And nobody knows the ball like Liz Gilles. *101 Ways to Work Out on the Ball* gives you exercises that will strengthen, lengthen, tone, and stretch your body like no other form of exercise can. The moves will work for beginners, intermediate, and advanced exercisers; some even require weights to sculpt your arms and legs while strengthening your core. The program includes workout plans and tips for progressing through the series.

Liz Gilles develops and stars in numerous videos including *Zone Pilates*, *Stability Ball Workouts*, *Stability Ball for Dummies*, and most recently her own "Core Fitness" line of videos. She is the owner and artistic director of The Insidescoop Pilates studios in New York, where she has been certifying teachers in the Pilates Method since 1997. She is regularly featured in news programs and national publications.